AF504365

David GIQUELLO

Chronic Diseases,

Avoid the 5 BIG killers!

Cancers

Cardio-Vasculars

Dementias

Diabetes

Depressions

Reference site for this book: www.veryveryhealthy.com
Pocket paper version ISBN: 978-2-9571628-1-9

© David GIQUELLO. All rights of reproduction, adaptation and translation, in whole or in part, reserved for all countries. The author is the sole owner of the rights and responsible for the content of this book.
© Royalty free cover photo, from pexels.com

Content

Warning

This book aims to share information and personal experiences on health and diet. This book does not in any way replace a medical consultation or the advice of any other health professional. Only your general practitioner or specialist is authorized to establish a medical diagnosis and prescribe the appropriate treatment resulting therefrom.

The use of the information provided in this book is under the full and entire responsibility of the user. Under no circumstances may the author or publisher of this book be held responsible for this use, as well as for errors, inaccuracies or omissions that may be presented therein.

According to Articles 10 of the European Convention on Human Rights of 4 November 1950 and 11 of the Charter of Fundamental Rights of the European Union of 2000: "Everyone has the right to freedom of expression. This right includes the freedom of opinion and the freedom to receive or communicate information or ideas without there being any interference from public authorities and without consideration of borders…"□

Dedication and thanks

I dedicate this book to all beings of good will, who act sincerely for peace and harmony. My thanks go to the many doctors and journalists who have published books and articles for decades to warn us of the importance of food and alternative medical solutions that exist, but which are unknown to the largest number.

My motivation for writing this book is service to others, to help all the sick and rebellious pacifists who are making efforts to improve the human and animal condition. The life of these volunteers is the most important factor for the future, because without those who are active in the community, nothing will change, and their good health and longevity are therefore essential to give every chance to a new era of joy, health and peace to see the light of day.

Yes, unfortunately, we are also lied to on the subject of health, as on the subject of alternative energy sources, the origin of humanity and its history, our physiological and psychological constitution, as well as on the nature of consciousness itself.

Can I advise you to go to a bookstore to find the many serious works on those many important subjects? The citizens of our modern countries read a lot of books, but why 90% of them are fictions and novels, when there are non-fiction works that deal with all these subjects essential to sustainable development, through an awareness of realities not addressed in our daily activities.

Today in 2020, thousands of useful books exist in our bookstores and libraries. Thanks to their authors who made the necessary efforts to share their discoveries and understandings. Researchers, investigative journalists, intelligent authors have gone to great lengths to publish information that can help us solve problems of all kinds that we face, so let's show them appreciation by buying their books and reading them to educate ourselves on subjects useful to us personally, but also to our community.

Let's make a difference and make 90% of the books purchased to be books providing practical and useful information, and keep 10% for our entertainment. After all, would we need as much to escape in a book if we were happy and healthy, integrated in a peaceful and balanced society, exchanging and laughing on a daily basis?

Thank you for purchasing this book as it will allow me to pay my bills and give me the time to work on other books that cover other important topics. ☐

Introduction

This book presents information which makes it possible to avoid the vast majority of diseases, and can be followed with confidence, since it comes from health professionals and scientific researchers.

This book integrates essential data from more than 25 different books, which I encourage you to buy and read in full, of which 19 authors are medical practicing doctors, 6 are doctors of science (PhD), and 2 are graduate nutritionists and dietitians working in hospitals.

I wanted to integrate more books written by women doctors, but I could not find the books that corresponded to the purpose of this book. I started with a review of hundreds of books on the subject of health, I selected more than 150, including 90 written by doctors, and only then did I choose in priority those which had the greatest potential to save lives and bring people back to good health, while being written by medical professionals. In addition to these books, which already exceed 7,000 pages, other information comes from publications by other doctors who have not written books.

I appeal to your indulgence on the possible faults and errors present in this book, because from the idea of this book to its publication, I gave myself 90 days, and a maximum of 400 pages, myself doing all the stages of selection, writing, correction, editing and graphics, for lack of financial resources on the one hand, but above all for the sake of speed, since each stage delegated to a professional would have added weeks or months of waiting, which seemed unnecessary to me, given the seriousness of the subject and the urgency of sharing these messages, gathered in a single book, since they can literally save lives, and get people out of situations of chronic suffering.

This book therefore deals with the main causes of current mortality and suffering. For each case I show the information and statistics presented on the official websites, then I share the information from several books of doctors who explain where the problems come from, and what to do to avoid them.

And after a conclusion in three parts, I kept the last pages of the book for suggestions on taking action, so that this section is easily accessible in everyday life, the time to integrate the different elements. I sincerely hope that this information will be useful to you and allow you to improve your general state of well-being☐

The reference books

The list of books which are the basis of this work, more than 25 titles, of which 19 authors are medical doctors, 2 qualified nutritionists, and 6 doctors in science (PhD). Other works by doctors and professors are cited, but in a shorter way.

1 - André Marie-Laure, nutritionist in hospital, French book "Preventing vascular accidents through food", from 2016, ISBN 978-2889117680

2 - Beljanski Mirko, Doctor of Science (PhD), French book "Cancer: the Beljanski approach" , from 2011, ISBN 978-2813202284

3 - Cathcart Robert, MD, book "MD on Vitamin C - 30,000 Patients", from 2018, ISBN 978-3746047058

4 - Cordain Loren, MD, book "The paleo diet: The diet without transformed food", from 2015, ISBN 978-2013964548

5 - Curtay Jean-Paul, MD, French book "Fibromyalgia, a global program to improve your health ", from 2011, ISBN 978-2916878829 6/7

6-7 - De Lorgeril Michel, MD, and Patricia Salen, nutritionist, French book "Preventing heart attacks and strokes", from 2011, ISBN 978-2916878881, and French book "The new Mediterranean diet. To protect your health and the planet ", from 2017, ISBN 978-2501111898

8 - Desaulniers Véronique, MD, French book "Heal Breast Cancer Naturally: 7 Essential Steps", from 2019, ISBN 978-1090881793

9 - Greger Michael, MD, and his team of volunteer doctors, book "Eating better can save your life", from 2018, ISBN 978-2266285155 (old title: "How not to die")

10 - Lagacé Jacqueline, Doctor of Science (PhD), French book "How I Overcame Pain and Chronic Inflammation Through Food", from 2011, ISBN 978-2365490443

11 - Levy Thomas, MD, book "The Original Panacea - Vitamin C", from 2017, ISBN 978-2879090214 , and book "Hidden Epidemic: Silent Oral Infections Cause Most Heart Attacks and Breast Cancers", from 2017, ISBN 978-0983772873

12 - Mosley Michael, MD, book "8 weeks to end diabetes without medication", from 2017, ISBN 979-1028503123.

13 - Mousseau Normand, Doctor of Science (PhD), book "How I conquered diabetes without medication", from 2016, ISBN 978-2365492065

14 - Nehls Michael, MD, French book "Cure alzheimer", from 2017, ISBN 978 -2330072834.

15 - Packer Lester, Doctor of Science (PhD), book "The Antioxidant Miracle: Your Complete Plan for Total Health and Healing", from 1999, ISBN 978-1620456194

16 - Pauling Linus, Doctor of Science (PhD), and Cameron Erwan, MD, book "Cancer and Vitamin C: A Discussion of the Nature, Causes, Prevention, and Treatment of Cancer With Special Reference to the Value of Vitamin C", 1993, ISBN 978-0940159211

17 - Rath Matthias, MD, book "Why animals don't have a heart attack… men do!", Of 2009, ISBN 978-9076332550

18 - Rath Matthias and Niedzwiecki Alexandra, MDs, book "Victory over cancer - Cancer The end of a disease of civilization - Book I - Scientific breakthrough", from 2011, ISBN 978-9076332826

19 - Ricard Matthieu, Doctor of Science (PhD), and Wolf Singer, MD, book "Brain & Meditation", from 2018, ISBN 978-2266279048

20/21 - Roques Jacques, MD, French book "Discovering EMDR (Personal development and accompaniment)", from 2012, ISBN 978-2729612153, and French book "Healing with EMDR. Treatment, theory, testimonies", of 2007, ISBN 978-2020881241.

22/23/24 - Schwartz Laurent, MD, French book "The end of diseases?" of 2019, ISBN 979-1020907059, French book "Cancer: A simple and nontoxic treatment" of 2016, ISBN 978-2365491778, French book "Cancer - Healing all the sick?" of 2013, ISBN 978-2755611472

25 - Seignalet Jean, MD, French book "Food or third medicine", of 2012, ISBN 978-2268074009

26 - Simoncini Tullio, MD, book "Cancer is a Fungus: A Revolution in Tumor Therapy ", of 2007, ISBN 978-8887241082

27 - Stone Irwin and Klenner Frederick Robert, MDs, "80 Years of High-Dose-Vitamin C Research", of 2018, ISBN 978-3752812756□

The main causes of death

This chapter establishes the list of the main causes of death, from data collected on the official website of the French Ministry of Health for local data, as well as the site of the European Union, then of the World Health Organization. Each cause of death and the means of prevention discovered by these doctors will then be dealt with in detail in the following chapters.

Statistics at the global level tend to be more and more similar in all countries, since humanity is migrating to the new type of modern, urban, sedentary and industrial life. It's living in the city in the midst of air pollution, working stressfully all day, and eating ultra-processed products without nutrients, which is becoming the norm for the majority of our human siblings.

Yet this was not the case only 100 years ago, or even less in remote places. Our bodies have not had time to adapt to such radical changes, which explains the explosion of these so-called "civilization diseases", incurable and inevitable…

Inevitable? Incurable? Really? However, numerous scientific studies show that they can be avoided by changing lifestyle, without drugs!

According to this information, it can be concluded that the major causes of death, excluding infections, are in order of magnitude:

1- Stroke and heart attack (grouped under the term Cardio-Vascular Diseases, or CVD)
2- Cancers
3- Dementias
4 - Diabetes / Obesity
5- Depressions / Suicides

It emerges from the following data that the general situation of the world population is in decline, despite technological advances and the increase in the number of hospitals and medical budgets. The modern lifestyle is definitely not compatible with our organisms, when it is based on the means we use today, combustion of hydrocarbons for the supply of energy, and massive use of chemicals for agriculture and food production.

Note on air pollution: It has become an important source of mortality, and a major official concern at the global level, since it strongly impacts health in general, and even more than smoking.

According to the French Ministry of Health:

https://solidarites-sante.gouv.fr/

The intensity of environmental exposures in the general population (air quality, water, endocrine disruptors, etc.) is lower than that of professional exposures, but they concern a very large number of people. In particular, air pollution is responsible for 48,000 deaths per year.

And according to the WHO, air pollution is the main environmental health risk worldwide. Thus, exposure to outdoor and indoor air pollution leads to premature death each year (we speak of premature death because exposure to air pollution shortens life) for approximately 6.5 million people around the world.

Causes of death in France

What the website of the French Ministry says, which has many pages on health, but very poorly organized for effective navigation. Source: https://solidarites-sante.gouv.fr/systeme-de-sante-et-medico-social/strategie-nationale-de-sante/article/la-strategie-nationale-de-sante-2018-2022

The national health strategy constitutes the framework for health policy in France. It is defined by the Government and is based on the analysis drawn up by the High Council of Public Health on the state of health of the population, its main determinants, as well as on the possible action strategies.

It reaffirms the principle carried by the World Health Organization, according to which health must be an objective of all public policies carried out in France and in the world. It aims to respond to the major challenges facing our health system, in particular those identified by the report of the High Council for Public Health:
-    health risks linked to the foreseeable increase in exposure to pollutants and toxic substances;
-    the risks of exposure of the population to the risks of infection;
-    chronic diseases and their consequences;
-    adapting the health system to demographic, epidemiological and societal challenges.

The latest report on the state of health of the French is here:
https://drees.solidarites-sante.gouv.fr/etudes-et-statistiques/publications/recueils-ouvrages-et-rapports/recueils-annuels/I- The state of population health / article / The state of health of the population in France Report 2017

However, the statistics are quite old, from 2013, in a report from 2017, when we are in 2020. Enough to be disappointed, considering that health should be the priority subject of the authorities, the least of things would be to have recent data.

Extracts from the summary: https: // drees. solidarites-sante.gouv.fr/IMG/pdf/synthese-2.pdf

"The reduction in mortality concerns most chronic diseases: between 1980 and 2012, mortality from all cancers (first cause of death) decreased by 1,5% on average per year for men and 1% for women."

Which means that in 32 years and hundreds of billions spent on chemicals, 1% less die from cancer, which is to say that nothing has changed!

"Between 2000 and 2013, the age-on-death rate from stroke decreased by 37.1%. This decrease is observed for both sexes, in those under 65 as well as in those over 65."

They show much better results against cardiovascular diseases, but well below the 80% reduction possible by changing the food of the French. Not to mention the tens of thousands of new paralyzed each year from stroke:

"Of the 567,000 deaths observed in mainland France in 2013, cancers and cardiovascular diseases are the most common causes (27.6% and 25.1% respectively), followed by diseases of the respiratory system (other than cancer), which represent one death in fifteen, and violent deaths (suicide, accidents, etc.) which also represent one death in fifteen."

"If mortality from stroke has been decreasing since the 2000s, the incidence of hospitalized patients has been increasing among those under 65 since 2002 and has tended to stabilize among those 65 and over since 2008."

A general deteriorating health, on problems which are easy to avoid according to many doctors:

"Hospitalizations for exacerbation of chronic obstructive pulmonary disease (COPD) increased between 2000 and 2014."

"The prevalence of pharmacologically treated diabetes increased by 4, 4% in 2010 to 4.7% in 2013 or around 3 million people, an increase which affects the over and under 65s of both sexes."

"The number of people affected by one or more of these diseases is constantly increasing. More worryingly, the increase in the frequency of chronic diseases also affects people under the age of 65 and especially women."

"Globally, the WHO considers that five of the ten most worrying pathologies in the 21st century are related to mental disorders: schizophrenia, bipolar disorder, addiction, depression and obsessive compulsive disorder. They are responsible for the major part of suicide mortality, severe disabilities and handicaps as well as a deteriorated quality of life for those affected."

"The number of people suffering from neurodegenerative pathologies will increase in the coming years. Alzheimer's disease and other dementias (MAAD) are a public health issue in all developed countries today."

Smoking is a scourge, as is alcohol abuse:
"The significant drop in smoking among men, observed for several decades until 2005, resulted in a 15% drop in rates standardized deaths linked to malignant tumors of the larynx, trachea, bronchi and lung, between 2002 and 2013. However, this rate increased by 39% among women over the same period; in total, daily smoking decreased by 2% for both sexes combined."

"Excessive alcohol consumption is also the cause of a significant proportion of morbidity (cancers, chronic liver diseases, mental disorders, after-effects of accidents) and premature mortality. Alcohol consumption has been decreasing steadily in France for several decades. Thus, France no longer occupies the top of the European ranking as it has long been the case, even if it remains in the group of the most consuming countries."

We really eat too much and badly in France:
"Half of adults are now overweight and, among these, one in six adults suffers from obesity."

And we burn too many non-renewable fuels:
"In particular, pollution by fine PM2.5 particles emitted by human activities is the cause each year, in mainland France, of at least 48,000 premature deaths (or 9 % of mortality in France)."

And it is always the poor who suffer the most:
"It is often the same populations, the least advantaged (low income, poorly qualified), who accumulate exposures to different risk factors for health, in the professional environment (exposure to work physically strenuous, working at night, with toxic products, etc.) or family (noise, poor air or water quality, etc.). They are also those whose behaviors (eating, physical activity, prevention, etc.) are the least favorable to health."

And to finish, we make in our old age, the fortune of the manufacturers of pills, and we end up dying from it:
"As a corollary to poly pathology, polypharmacy, usual and often justified, poses significant risks to health, especially in the elderly. International literature has shown that there is indeed a significant association between polypharmacy and the occurrence of adverse effects, drug interactions, falls, or even increased mortality. In 2013, 40% of people aged 75 and over were affected by cumulative polypharmacy, i.e. they accumulate on average 10 or more drugs over 3 months and 33% take more than 10 drugs continuously."

Causes of death in Europe

Information from the official E.U. site, for 2015.
Source: https://ec.europa.eu/eurostat/statistics-
explained/index.php?title=Causes_of_death_statistics/en the

- Leading cause of death in Europe, cardiovascular disease with more than 2.6 million deaths.
- Second cause, cancers with more than 1.7 million.
- In third respiratory diseases with 0.45 million, mainly suffered by people over 65 years of age.
- Nervous diseases, dementia among others, with 0.2 million.
- Suicides, with 55,000 deaths.
- Transport accidents, 30,000 deaths.

(figures rounded, based on 500 million Europeans in 2015)

Selected extracts: "The latest estimated information on causes of death in the EU-28 relates to the reference period 2015. Table 1 shows that diseases of the circulatory system and cancer (malignant tumors) were by far the main causes of deaths in the European Union."

"After diseases of the circulatory system and cancer, respiratory diseases were the third leading cause of death in the EU-28 in 2015, with an average of 88 deaths per 100,000 inhabitants. In this disease category, chronic conditions of the lower respiratory tract were the leading cause of death, followed by pneumonia. Respiratory diseases are age-related, with a large majority of deaths occurring in people aged 65 and over."

"Among people under the age of 65, the main causes of death differed somewhat in their relative importance (see Table 2). Cancer was the leading cause of death in this age group, followed by diseases of the circulatory system. Diseases of the respiratory system were not among the top three causes of death for this category." End of extracts

Causes of death worldwide

Information from the official website of the World Health Organization, for 2016: Source from WHO May 24, 2018 https://www.who.int/fr/news-room/fact- sheets / detail / the-top-10-causes-of-death

The main causes of death:
1. Leading cause of death in the world, cardiovascular diseases with more than 15 million deaths.
2. Second cause, respiratory diseases with 7.5 million.
3. Third, dementia with 2 million.
4. Fourth, lung, throat and tracheal cancers 1.5 million.
5. Diabetes mellitus 2 million.
6. Road accidents 1.5 million.
7. Diarrheal diseases 1.5 million.

Selected extracts: "Of the 56.9 million deaths that occurred worldwide in 2016, more than half (54%) is due to the following 10 causes. Ischemic heart disease and stroke are the leading causes of death worldwide, responsible for a total of 15.2 million deaths in 2016. They have remained the leading causes of death in the world for the past 15 years."

"Chronic obstructive pulmonary disease caused 3 million deaths in 2016, while lung cancer (with those of the trachea and bronchi) caused 1.7 million deaths. Diabetes killed 1.6 million people in 2016, compared to less than a million in 2000. Deaths from dementia more than doubled between 2000 and 2016, making it the 5th leading cause of death in the world in 2016 when they only came in 14th position in 2000."

"More than half of the deaths in low-income countries in 2016 were due to so-called "Group I" diseases, communicable diseases, maternal causes, pathologies occurring during pregnancy and childbirth and nutritional deficiencies. In contrast, they account for only 7% of deaths in high-income countries. Lower respiratory tract infections were among the leading causes of death in all income groups."

"Non-communicable diseases (NCDs) account for 71% of deaths worldwide, ranging from 37% in low-income countries to 88% in high-income countries. Of the 10 causes of death, all but one are NCDs in high-income countries. In absolute numbers of deaths, however, 78% of deaths from NCDs worldwide have occurred in low- and middle-income countries."

"Trauma claimed 4.9 million lives in 2016, more than a quarter (29%) of which were due to road traffic crashes."□

1. Preventing Cardiovascular Diseases

All Cardiovascular Diseases (CVD) are the leading cause of death worldwide.

A / "Official Speech" summarizes what the medical authorities say, as well as a book summarizing known means of prevention, written by a graduate nutritionnist.

B / "The Rath theory" presents the book by Doctor Rath, who participated in the work of the double Nobel Prize winner Pr Linus Pauling, and together had established the Rath / Pauling theory which would be the solution to CVD. The seriousness of the speakers and the theory should prompt us to try it on a large-scale scientific study, since it would prevent CVD in any situation, regardless of a change in diet and lifestyle.

C / "Lyon Study" presents one of the books by Doctor de Lorgeril, who was the main investigator of the famous "Lyon Heart study" which scientifically proved the remarkable effectiveness of the adoption of a traditional Mediterranean type diet against CVD.

D / "Super Nutrition" concerns the book by Doctor Greger, who with his team of volunteer doctors, reviews hundreds of scientific publications every week, and publishes summaries on multiple medical subjects or food, and their repercussions on health.

Enough to understand clearly that a change in nutrition is essential to be healthy and avoid these devastating CVDs.☐

A / CVD, the official discourse

CVD according to the WHO

Source: https://www.who.int/health-topics/cardiovascular-diseases/#tab=tab_1

Cardiovascular disease (CVD) is the leading cause of death in the world, killing 17.9 million people each year, about 31% of all deaths worldwide.

85% of all CVD deaths are due to heart attacks (Myocardial Infarction, MI) and strokes, and one third of these deaths occur prematurely in people under the age of 70.

Cardiovascular disease is a group of disorders of the heart and blood vessels and includes coronary artery disease, cerebrovascular disease, rheumatic heart disease and other conditions.

People at risk for CVD may have increased blood pressure, glucose and lipids, as well as being overweight and obese.

CVD according to the French Ministry of Health

Source: https://solidarites-sante.gouv.fr/soins-et-maladies/maladies/maladies-cardiovasascular/article/maladies-cardiovasascular

Last update 14.05.19, (more than 7 months ago. It may be a part-time job to fight the second cause of death ...)

On this page cardiovascular problems are well listed, and the causes listed correspond to what science has discovered. No problem at this level, very good diagnosis. It is at the level of the actions to be taken as an individual that I remain on my need. I guess I just have to go to my doctor to get prescribed pills that will control my health problems ... And why not encourage and offer visits to qualified nutritionists, who will explain how science discovered how to prevent up to 80% of these cardiovascular problems?

Ah yes, but this is done without the need for drugs, so apart from the vegetable farmers no one would gain from this prevention by changing their lifestyle... And the pills from our industrial pharmaceutical flagships, who will buy them if 4 out of 5 patients are cured??

Selected extracts: "Cardiovascular or cardio-neurovascular diseases are the leading cause of death in the world, the second in France (the first for women) just after cancer. Despite four decades of reduced mortality and morbidity thanks to prevention and therapeutic progress, cardio-neurovascular diseases remain the cause of around 140,000 deaths per year; they are also one of the main causes of morbidity with 3.5 million people (insured under the general scheme) treated in 2012, and more than 11 million for vascular risk or diabetes."

"The most common mechanism of cardio-neurovascular disease is atherosclerosis, by building up a fatty deposit on the internal walls of the blood vessels supplying these organs."

"The main risk factors for cardio-neurovascular disease are linked to lifestyle: smoking, unbalanced diet, lack of physical activity, harmful use of alcohol, psychosocial factors such as stress."

"Preventing smoking, facilitating a balanced diet and the consumption of fruits and vegetables, regular physical activity, and avoiding the harmful use of alcohol can reduce the risk of cardiovascular disease."

"Reducing this risk is based on reducing modifiable factors: factors linked to lifestyle habits (quitting smoking, adopting a balanced diet and reducing salt consumption, having regular physical activity and limiting physical inactivity, avoiding harmful use of alcohol, reducing stress, reducing overweight) and resort to medication if necessary for high blood pressure, diabetes, or high cholesterol."

So, it is a question of changing one's lifestyle, and only then, if still necessary, resorting to medication. So why is this not what health professionals do, why do we go directly to the "pills solution"?

Lack of staff, lack of time? And wouldn't the billions spent on pills be enough to recruit staff for education in good health and protective lifestyles?

Concerning strokes

90% of strokes are preventable by changing their lifestyle, according to this publication in the scientific journal The Lancet. And 30% to 40% of strokes, more or less a third, are attributable only to air pollution, especially PM 2.5 nanoparticles.

International study published in The Lancet in 2016:
https://www.thelancet.com/journals/laneur/article/PIIS1474-4422(16)30073-4/fulltext
Selected extracts: "Our results suggest that more than 90% of strokes are due to modifiable risk factors, and controlling behavioral and metabolic risk factors could prevent more than three-quarters of the global amount of stroke.

Air pollution has emerged as a significant contributor to the global burden of stroke, particularly in low and middle-income countries, and reducing exposure to air pollution should therefore be a top priority to reduce the burden of stroke in these countries.

We have established 17 risk factors:
- ambient pollution of particles,
- pollution of domestic air by solid fuels,
- exposure to lead,
- diet rich in sodium,
- diet rich in sugary drinks,
- diet low in fruits,
- diet low in vegetables,
- diet low in whole grains,
- alcohol consumption (any dose),
- low physical activity,
- smoking,
- passive smoking,
- high BMI,
- fasting plasma glucose,
- high SBP
- High total cholesterol
- low glomerular filtration rate (GFR)
- Air pollution concerns fine PM 2.5 particles from outdoor and domestic air." End of extracts

The French INSERM confirms the important role of pollution on its page dedicated to Cerebral Vascular Accidents
https://www.inserm.fr/information-en-sante/dossiers-information/accident-vasascular-cerebral-avc

"Pollution, particularly from the air, would also increase the risk of stroke. Several studies indicate that peaks in air pollution are correlated with an increase in hospitalizations for stroke and mortality from stroke."☐

80% of CVDs are avoidable

According to this state-certified nutritionist:

Mrs. Marie-Laure André, French book, "Preventing vascular accidents through food", from 2016, ISBN 978-2889117680

I added it to the chapter "Official Speech" since it is written by a French civil servant, dietician in a public hospital environment.

Summary of key points:

In the preface, doctor Jean-Michel Tartière, MD, head of the cardiovascular division, recalls that the "Mediterranean diet" is one of the cornerstones of our good health, and that it is a means of preventing cardiovascular illnesses.

The introduction reminds us that cardiovascular disease (CVD) was the second leading cause of death in France in 2015, after cancer, with more than 150,000 deaths per year! There are 110,000 myocardial infarctions per year in France.

Stroke is the third leading cause of death for men, and the first for women, and the leading cause of disability, with 130,000 per year!

We learn that the risk factors are clearly identified, and that many of these accidents could be avoided. From the beginning it is written that it is a certain lifestyle which allows to act directly on the risk factors. No need for miraculous products or high-tech machines, just a few habit changes. Junk food is singled out, which is progressing all over the world, despite a certain awareness on the part of the populations ...

This book puts us directly in the heart of the matter, with the means of prevention;

Extract from page 11: "This type of diet is the Mediterranean diet. Rich in fiber, antioxidant compounds, vegetable fats, and poor in animal fats and processed foods. More than a diet, it's an art of eating!" End of extract

High blood pressure, given as representing 35% of the risk of stroke, is discussed on page 33. It is clearly stated that it is due to the loss of elasticity of the arteries and to their stiffening. The solution is given on page 34, extract:

"High blood pressure is not inevitable: certain parameters such as physical activity and diet can significantly and durably lower blood pressure figures."

So here again, diet and physical activity are the solutions against the 40% risk of stroke due to hypertension.

Stress is discussed on page 46, as also a risk factor, but again no mention of the destructive biological processes caused by stress.

Other interesting topics are covered, such as excess weight and alcohol.

In the third part, page 60, she tackles the subject of the demonization of fats, which have been targets for decades. Our body needs fat, since all of our cells have membranes made of fat, and our brain is full of it too! There are also essential fatty acids, which our body needs, and which it can't manufacture on its own. So we have to eat fats.

Extract page 61: "In reality, there is no "bad fat" since all fatty acids, whether saturated or unsaturated, have an essential role in the organism."

Very important vitamins are also attached to these fats that we eat, which we cannot do without. On the other hand, synthetic fats are a problem, because unnatural, these so-called "hydrogenated" fats, are not recognized by the organism and its microbiota and cause harmful inflammatory reactions.

Page 64 is important because it reminds us that essential fatty acids must be absorbed in natural proportions. That is to say in the proportions presented by fish meat, where Omega-3 are more important. Modern processed foods are especially rich in omega 6, which in too large quantities causes inflammation. The proportion between these two types of fatty acids should be 1 to 5, or 5 times more omega 6, but modern food doubles this ratio, increasing to 1 to 10, which is far too much.

Then the Lyon Study, from INSERM in Bron, from 1994 to 1999 is mentioned, and one clearly reads this shocking fact, which should have been adopted by all French people since that date, that the adoption of a Mediterranean diet avoids up to 73% of relapsed heart attacks!!

But since this study, the number of cardiovascular accidents has continued to increase, which means that the information has not passed down, and many people die or suffer from it today in 2020, when the solution is scientifically known and verified for over 25 years!

This book then mentions some studies that have been done since, very few and especially less targeted, and never deepening the subject, like the PREDIMED study of 2013, which showed less encouraging results.

Fiber is discussed on p 69. It is still a compound that is absent from modern, industrial and processed food. Yet fibers are essential to the rate of transit in our intestines and are an important part of the food for the good bacteria of our microbiome which make so many essential micronutrients for us. Fiber is also needed to slow the spread of sugars and prevent dramatic spikes in blood sugar.

Of course, the fresh fruits and vegetables of the Mediterranean diet are rich in antioxidants of all kinds, vitamins, minerals and essential enzymes ... provided you do not cook them all and absorb a good quantity fresh.

Note that she forgot to mention air pollution as an important factor of stress on our circulatory system. Experts consider that the nanoparticles of exhaust gases and tires dust are responsible for 40% of strokes! Because these tiny molecules strongly irritate the walls of our arteries, after having easily penetrating thanks to their size, they go everywhere.

This book still gives lots of useful information, and even recipes to help novices find a healthy and more natural way of eating. The back cover contains a striking sentence that says it all:

"Strokes and heart attacks are not inevitable! You can limit their risks by 80% by adopting a healthy lifestyle."

And now, 80% fewer cardiovascular accidents, in France it would be 90,000 heart attacks and 105,000 strokes avoided each year.

Do these millions of victims worldwide know that their lives are turned upside down due to lack of information?

How can we make them aware of this information and take it seriously, to avoid this suffering?

B / Dr. Rath's treatment for CVD

I prefer this ambitious program, based on scientific results, to the imprecise little summary on the page of the Ministry of Health!

According to the book by Dr. Matthias Rath "Why animals do not have heart attack... but people do!", from 2009, ISBN 978-9076332550

All chapters are downloadable for free, select your language from the menu among 14 available: http://www.dr-rath-foundation.org/2018/07/why-animals-dont-get-heart-attacks-but-people-do/

"The time has come for humanity to eradicate heart attack, stroke, and other cardiovascular disease. Yesterday, the discovery of microorganisms, the cause of infectious diseases, made it possible to control epidemics. Today, discovering the effects of a long-term vitamin deficiency will help control cardiovascular disease, the leading cause of death and disability in the 21st century. Humanity is now able to eradicate them."

And from its second paragraph, the foundations are laid; that is, the problem comes from micronutrient deficiencies, caused by our modern foods that lack them, and the solution presented is the supplementation in these micronutrients, while waiting to improve our diet.

"Animals do not have heart attack because they make vitamin C which protects their vascular walls. In humans, unable to produce it, a deficiency weakens them. Cardiovascular disease is an early form of scurvy. Clinical studies have shown that daily and optimal consumption of essential vitamins and nutrients naturally stops the progression of cardiovascular disease and causes them to regress."

In the last century, science has uncovered solutions to infectious diseases, which were by far the biggest killers in the world. And soon after these same scientists also discovered the causes of non-infectious diseases, at least for the majority of them, but there, instead of a gradual eradication that one might have expected, it is an epidemic progression that takes place. Cardiovascular diseases, cancers, obesity, diabetes, dental cavities are exploding all over the world, when we know that they are directly the cause of poor nutrition.

Why, if we really cannot maintain humans in a healthy diet, we do not prescribe them the food supplements which would make it possible to eradicate the major part of these evils. Is it because pills that bring in a lot of money and keep humans active and productive for decades, when infectious diseases nailed them to bed and thus prevented the industrial model from developing?

Excerpt: "Natural prevention of disorders of blood circulation, infarctions, strokes, alterations of blood vessels in diabetes, hypertension, heart failure, heart rhythm disorders and many other problems with the circulatory system. This book documents the scientific breakthrough to end cardiovascular disease.

It is not too high cholesterol, but weakened artery walls that are the main cause of cardiovascular disease. This discovery made it possible, for the first time, to understand why millions of people suffer from myocardial infarction, but not from nose or ear infarction.

In this book, Dr. Rath, Linus Pauling's last close scientific collaborator, summarizes his revolutionary medical discoveries in scientific language accessible to all.

Dr. Rath's book has already been translated into all of the most widely spoken languages and read by millions of people. Many people immediately took advantage of these revolutionary discoveries to improve their health.

With the publication of this landmark book online, Dr. Rath is now taking another step to save millions of lives. If you've already read this book, you will consider Dr. Rath's goal of "Health for All by 2020" to be realistic and achievable."

The introduction states that this book provides advice to us and our family. Let him show us how to significantly extend our lives. It allows us to recover our health, and shows us how to act.

The program is in 10 steps:
- Becoming aware of the importance of the cardiovascular system
- Stabilizing the walls of our blood vessels
- Eliminating deposits from our arteries without surgery
- Relaxing the walls of these so-called blood vessels
- Optimizing our cardiac performance
- Protecting our cardiovascular system against aging
- Exercising regularly
- Eating a balanced diet
- Finding time for relaxation
- Acting now without waiting

Then he presents the thirty or so micronutrients that are important for the proper functioning of our cells. Vitamins, minerals, amino acids and trace elements.

Of course, many of these elements are present in an improved Mediterranean diet, but some such as vitamin C, really require supplementation to reach the advanced figures, except in summer maybe if we eat a lot of fresh fruits and vegetables.

The recommended amounts of minerals are minimal and are easily found in fresh green vegetable juices, for example.

Chapter 2 provides an update on cardiovascular disease, with many explanations, diagrams, photos and medical imaging results. In my opinion these are proves for any open-minded medical professional who would bother to study them. It addresses atherosclerosis, infarction and stroke. We immediately understand that it is a lack of building blocks of our cells that causes these health problems, and that the solutions exist:

"A selection of essential cellular nutrients makes it possible to stop cardiovascular diseases and reverse their course."

There are also testimonies written by cured patients, having had, quote, "phenomenal" results.

Next are presentations of the results of clinical studies that have taken place for decades, explanations that allow us to understand how well the positive results have been known in the last century, but ignored by the vast majority.

Page 55, a shorter list of supplements and their usefulness; Vitamins C, E, D, proline, lysine, folic acid, biotin, copper, chondroitin sulfate, N-Acetylglucosamine and pycnogenol.

Then he explains us "How does vitamin C prevent atherosclerosis?", and the problem of scurvy as a whole, from its early effects to its final phase. Later he presents irrefutable proof that atherosclerosis is caused by vitamin C deficiency. For this purpose they use guinea pigs, one of the rare mammals which do not produce vitamin C in their liver.

"Two groups of guinea pigs received exactly the same amounts of cholesterol, fat, protein, sugar, salt and other ingredients, with one exception: vitamin C. Group B received 60 mg of vitamin C per day, in proportion to the human weight. This amount represents the official recommended intake per person in most countries of the world. Group A, on the other hand, received 5,000 mg of vitamin C per day.

The illustration shows very clear differences between the arteries of the animals of the two groups. Group B animals (vitamin C deficiency) develop atheroma deposits (white areas), especially in areas close to the heart (right part of the image). The aorta of the animals in group A remained healthy and showed no deposit formation."

Guinea pigs who did not receive vitamin C in their diet, developed atherosclerosis, the others did not! The images are breathtaking. By the way, for all the guinea pig friends, think about their vitamin C if you want them to live longer.

In summary, the positive effects of essential cellular nutrients on atherosclerosis are:
- Stability of the arterial wall through optimal production of collagen.
- Decrease in the accumulation of muscle cells in the arterial wall.
- "Teflon" protection and regression of fatty deposits on the arterial walls.

The third chapter provides an update on cholesterol and other secondary risk factors, and how a selection of essential cellular nutrients can help people with fat metabolism disorders. Of course our diet will also determine the dose of cholesterol that will circulate in our blood, but also how much our body will manufacture. Let's not forget that cholesterol is an essential brick for the survival of our body, which is why it produces it all the time. There are also patient testimonials.

In fact, beyond the good or bad cholesterol, LDL or HDL, it is Lipoprotein(a), discovered in 1963, which plays the role of fat glue in the arteries, much more troublesome than cholesterol. Lipoprotein(a) is a secondary risk factor ten times more dangerous than cholesterol.

Many pages explain in detail the role of the different fat molecules linked to clogging of the arteries, and the role of the scapegoat that has been given to cholesterol since the last century, and the key dates of this propaganda are listed.

At the end of this chapter we find the list of specific nutrients for the treatment of fat metabolism disorders, and their specific roles. Vitamins C, E, D, B1, B2, B3, B5, B6, biotin, folic acid, and carnitine.

The fourth part concerns hypertension, which is given by official statistics as representing 40% of the risk of stroke. It contains the basic data relating to essential cellular nutrients in the treatment of hypertension.

"Essential cellular nutrients help lower hypertension naturally. They indeed protect the arterial walls and thus prevent atherosclerotic plaques from forming or developing; on the other hand, they decrease the tension on the arterial walls."

Coq-10 is mentioned there

"Scientific research and clinical studies have shown that magnesium and coenzyme Q-10 have a hypotensive effect. People with high blood pressure are advised to start taking essential cellular nutrients as soon as possible and to inform their doctor.

This program supplements the usual medication. Do not stop or change your medication without consulting your doctor."

Results of clinical studies are presented, as well as some testimonial letters sent by assisted patients. The specific essential cellular nutrients in the treatment of hypertension. See details in the book: Vitamin C, E, arginine, magnesium, calcium and bioflavonoids.

Chapters 5, 6 and 8 deal with heart problems, heart failure and heart rhythm disorders (Arrhythmia), angina pectoris, and the effects of cell medicine on these problems. With results of clinical studies and different products tested, more testimonials as in the other chapters.

Chapter 7 deals with diabetes and related cardiovascular diseases, which of course is an inflammatory factor in the walls of the circulatory system, because insulin is a very aggressive molecule. "Millions of Europeans suffer from a disturbance in the metabolism of sugars. Heart attack, stroke, and other circulatory disorders are among the most feared consequences of diabetes."

Chapter 9: Cardiovascular risks due to the environment, lifestyle and hereditary factors. Essential cellular nutrients help reduce cardiovascular risks due to the environment, lifestyle and hereditary factors such as:

- An unbalanced diet
- Smoking
- Stress
- Contraceptives
- Diuretics and other drugs
- Dialysis
- Surgical procedures
- Hereditary factors of cardiovascular risks

The tenth chapter explains in depth the proponents of Cellular Medicine developed by Doctor Rath and his team of doctors and scientists.

It is the summary of all the micronutrients, and their role(s) in the proper functioning of cells, and therefore of the organism. As well as a comparison of the therapeutic objectives and the effectiveness between traditional medicine and Cellular Medicine.

The following chapter is edifying, and explains to us why we do not have access to this intelligent medicine, mainly because the pharmaceutical industries are not interested in the tiny profits of the sale of food supplements and guidebooks on healthy food... it is sure that cancer treatments that bring in tens of thousands of euros per year and per patient are enormously more profitable!

So, again the same conclusion with Doctor Rath, we are lied to and left to die in suffering for reasons of financial interests!

The last chapter reminds us of the stages in history that led to the concept of Cellular Medicine.

The historic conference of Dr Rath in May 4, 2002 at Stanford University

Clinical studies: naturally reversing the course of cardiovascular disease is possible

The Rath / Pauling patent against cardiovascular diseases

Dr Matthias Rath with the support of Pr Linus Pauling, received a patent in 1994 for a method which consists in removing the plaques of lipoproteins which obstruct the cardiovascular system, without surgery. It's within everyone's reach, and it immediately stops the process of obstructing veins and arteries. Professor Pauling explained that this weakening of the arterial walls is the chronic (long-term) form of scurvy.

The WHO recommended dose of 60 mg of vitamin C per day can prevent the acute (urgent) form of scurvy, but not the chronic form, which causes the body to gradually disintegrate, the arteries being weakened and blocked over the years. Taking megadoses of vitamin C immediately stops this process of clogging of the arteries and vice versa, and little by little they are liberated from the lipoproteins which clog them. The addition of lysine to megadoses of vitamin C greatly accelerates the unclogging process, lysine attaching to lipoproteins to evacuate them in the stool. You will see the difference in the first weeks of this diet!

You can view and print this patent here: US5278189A, United States. Prevention and treatment of occlusive cardiovascular disease with ascorbate and substances that inhibit the binding of lipoprotein(a)
https://patents.google.com/patent/US5278189A/en

Abstract: The invention relates to a method of preventing and treating cardiovascular diseases, such as atherosclerosis, by administering therapeutically effective doses of a medicament comprising ascorbate, lipoprotein(a) binding inhibitors and antioxidants. What is claimed is:

Pharmaceutical composition consisting essentially of ascorbate, tranexamic acid, lysine and nicotinic acid, said ingredients in an amount effective for treating occlusive cardiovascular diseases associated with Lp(a). A method of treating occlusive cardiovascular disease comprising the step of administering to a subject a therapeutic composition comprising ascorbate and tranexamic acid in an amount sufficient to decrease the binding of lipoprotein(a) to the walls of blood vessels.□

C / CVDs according to Dr. de Lorgeril

According to Dr. de Lorgeril's book "Preventing a heart attack and stroke", from 2011, ISBN 978-2916878881

Book co-written between the doctor and researcher at the CNRS in Lyon, Michel de Lorgeril, and Patricia Salen, nutritionist and research assistant in Grenoble, France. Dr de Lorgeril was the principal investigator in the Lyon Heart Study of the 1990s, and Ms. Salen was responsible for the nutrition part.

As a reminder, the Lyon Heart study, during the years 1980-90, had for the first time rigorously demonstrated the protective effect of adopting a traditional Mediterranean diet, with up to 73% less relapse of heart attack and therefore also increased longevity.

This book is therefore a scientific reference on the subject of the prevention of cardiovascular diseases and cancers through food. Deepening of these discoveries should have been carried out by the medical authorities responsible for the health of their citizens, but this was not the case, and moreover classical reasons are given in this book, such as the powerful lobbying of the pharmaco industries and medical professionals who do not wish to lose market share even in return for the well-being of populations.

The first part concerns the prevention of myocardial infarction, the leading cause of death in France and worldwide. Cardiovascular accidents (stroke) being the third cause after cancers. The introduction tells us that although complicated to explain or understand, cardiovascular disease is easy to prevent, and this book tells us how to do it. Even in France, where help arrives quickly and is very well organized, trained and equipped, another 50% of infarction victims die within an hour. In some fragile populations, the death rate at a few days may even rise to 80%.

Unfortunately, doctors do not have training in nutrition, nor the time to explain the long tunings to their patients, and the shortcut is generally to use drugs, without any explanation of the well-known prevention possibilities which are very effective.

Air pollution also has a large part in the occurrence of cardiovascular diseases, by the inflammation generated by micro and nanoparticles, such as those coming from exhaust pipes, wood heating or urban power stations, and industries. (But also dust from tires rubbing on the road)

Eating habits are of course the basic terrain for prevention. In particular the deficiencies accumulated over the years due to foods too low in micronutrients or processed and made indigestible.

Physical exercise is also essential, because a sedentary lifestyle is not natural for humans who have always had active days.

In Chapter 3 they present the ultimate proves that it is our way of life that must be improved to prevent these diseases, and not hope that some special foods or supplements will change our lives in a miraculous way.

This book presents conclusions based on the findings of the Lyon study, and others that were then carried out by other groups of doctors and scientists. These are not speculations or experiments in tubes, but facts which have been verified on living people. It is a complicated story that led to the implementation of the Lyon study, but which is completely revealed in this book. To sum it up, the Lyon cardiology center was the only one that did not change the lifestyle of patients after a heart transplant. And this led to high death rates, since patients remained sedentary, drank too much, smoked and lived as before their heart problems occurred. And it is thanks to this situation that they were able to see that a change in diet and lifestyle changed the game, and allowed patients to live much longer. It was a combination of exceptional circumstances and characters, as is often the case in science and elsewhere, that led to these incredible scientific discoveries and proves.

The lifestyle corrections were simple:
- Stop smoking
- Alcohol, only wine during meals
- Traditional Mediterranean diet
- Organized physical exercise

Cholesterol was not a factor that changed the results. Because the lesions of atherosclerosis were of a very large variety, and that it would be nonsense to attribute this to cholesterol. One more thing learned and proven for good thanks to this study!

Chapter 4 concerns the formidable discoveries of the Lyon study. The participants in this study were Dr Michel de Lorgeril, Patricia Salen, the Director of INSERM Serge Renaud, the Head of Department of the Cardiological Hospital of Lyon Pr Jacques Delaye, Pr André-Fouet, Pr Beaune, the Pr Delahaye, Pr Froment, Pr Normand, Pr Touboul, as well as Professors Epstein, Ducimetière, Nordoy, Rutishauser, Righetti, and Doctors Paillard and Guidollet.

The Lyon Diet Heart Study was designed in the 1980s, and the goal was to find out how to reduce the production of clotting platelets in the body to fight against clots in the arteries. They thought that decreasing platelet activity could be a solution.

Epidemiologists had previously presented the Mediterranean (especially the Greeks) and the Japanese as having less cardiovascular disease. The Mediterranean nutritional model was therefore adopted because it was easier to accept and implement in France. Changing people's eating habits is very difficult, and they were inspired by the work of Paul Watzlavick and Milton Erickson to do so. It was discovered that this diet had no effect on platelet activity, but large effects on health in general.

Patients had to lower their intake of animal products and their fats in order to lower cholesterol levels. That is to say, less fatty meats and cold meats, almost no eggs, fatty seafood products not recommended, even fatty fish, and even almonds, nuts and peanuts, as well as avocados were not recommended. It was not possible to advise drinking more red wine, for ethical reasons, although they are now convinced that this would have further improved the results.

The goal was to stay just below, at 35% fat in the daily calorie total, so as not to restrict the participants too much. For those who did not like olive oil, they could take rapeseed oil.

To sum up, it was a question of eating: less animal products, meats, cold meats and dairy products, and more plant products, fruits, vegetables, legumes, and cereals.

All the details on this "modernized Mediterranean diet" are on page 255.

Main results of the Lyon Heart Study

With the positive pre-results, they received pressure to publish everything immediately, but that would have ended the test, and the group fought to be able to continue even after the removal of financial support, in order to complete the study and have more convincing and consolidated results over the medium term of several additional years. The final analysis was published in 1999.

This study showed that by switching to a traditional Mediterranean diet, patients reduced by 50 to 70% their risks of having a cardiovascular accident, be it infarction, stroke, or heart failure, and there was less mortality too. No treatment, even today, has shown such preventive effectiveness. It's a major discovery!

Fortunately, this study has been cited thousands of times since then and has inspired many more studies around the world. The modern notion of nutrition as prevention of CVD and cancer started from there. A dozen studies have since been initiated on various populations, with similar results, fewer illnesses and a longer life expectancy. Nevertheless, the results would have been even better if all the participants had followed the nutritional advice given more precisely, and if some had not been in the terminal phase of life before the start of the trial. Some had very damaged hearts from previous heart attacks.

Many patients had nutritional deficiencies, deficiencies of essential fatty acids or amino acids, group B vitamins or vitamin C, or minerals and trace elements like selenium. And the larger the deficits, the more serious the heart problems. To summarize, to have good heart muscles you need to have enough selenium and vitamin C. This has been proven to be very important for heart function.

But today no doctor or cardiologist is looking for the possible deficiencies of their patients in vitamin C or selenium. In 2011, a large epidemiological study on 20,000 people highlighted the lack of vitamin C and the risks of heart failure, confirming their discovery more than 10 years earlier. But our vascular system is also important, and especially the good health of its internal wall, the endothelium, and of biological systems which depend on our nutrition.

Later, in the chapter on heart attack he explains how to make one's own heart resistant. There are at least 3 known means for this:
- Moderate physical exercise
- Less alcohol consumption
- Consumption of certain plant polyphenols
- Omega-3s also strengthen the health of the heart muscle.

Following are explanations on the formation of clots which lead to myocardial infarction. This clot formation is directly linked to lifestyle. For example, meat contains a fatty acid, called arachidonic, made from omega-6 linoleic acid, which increases the activity of the platelets that form clots. The omega-3 / omega-6 ratio is crucial to maintain the balance between thinning and coagulation of blood, and it is not complicated to maintain it at the right balance, since it is precisely what is found in the Mediterranean Diet!

He recalls that cholesterol plays no role in the activity of clotting platelets. These serve to block cuts or cracks in the arterial wall, and therefore do not return to function until after an attack on this wall, by a toxic substance, such as the elements of cigarette smoke for example. After coagulation a more solid structure is formed, the fibrin, filaments which enclose the platelets and stick them against the wall, and the clot begins its formation as well.

Smokers and diabetics have higher levels of fibrinogen than others, the molecule that makes fibrin filaments. Those who exercise or who consume wine moderately during meals, on the contrary have less fibrinogen. Nicotine stimulates the secretion of adrenaline which in turn stimulates the activity of platelets, and the carbon monoxide present in smoke is a real attacker on the walls of the arteries. A real anti-health cocktail!

Chapter 4 on cholesterol is important, because 7 million of French people consume cholesterol-lowering drugs, while the theory is false. Anti cholesterol treatments are as useless as harmful, he tells us, and he advises us to read his book "Cholesterol, lies and propaganda", as well as the books on the subject, by Thierry Souccar editions.

He then explains in detail 2 theories on atherosclerosis. He mentions lipoprotein(a) in an insert, but does not refer to the work of Dr. Matthias Rath and Pr. Linus Pauling and their discoveries and publications on the subject. To the question, "why does Lp(a) promote thrombosis?", he replies that it interferes with fibrinolysis by reducing its activity, and thus promotes the formation of solid and obstructive clots. He mentions a parallelism between Lp(a) and cholesterol, both being similarly high in patients. He points out that experts generally ignore this guilty Lp(a), and not cholesterol which plays no role in coagulation, nor in the biology of platelets or in fibrinolysis.

Chapter 5 deals with stroke, which does not only happen to the elderly, since a third of the victims are under 65 years of age. Hemorrhagic strokes representing at least 40% of all strokes. Many drugs promote hemorrhagic strokes, such as statins and thinners. It seems that the atherosclerosis observed in the cerebral arteries is different from that of the coronary arteries, because those of the brain are of different constitution, having no muscular capacity for spasmodic contraction.

The third part of the book deals with conventional risk factors for infarction and stroke. An insert on tobacco is particularly interesting because it mentions the toxicity of carbon monoxide as being particularly aggressive for the walls of the arteries.

In my opinion, this parallels the explanations of Dr Laurent Schwartz who discovered during his research on the harmfulness of cigarettes for tobacco manufacturers, that the most dangerous was the CO2 sucked in when smoking, from combustion. Indeed, these two gases are acidifying, as is well known in ecological circles, since we hear all the time that the oceans become more acidic from absorbing CO2 from the atmosphere.

Our body being mainly water, and our cells bathing in a matrix of water and collagen, we can imagine the harm that these gases can do to us, by acidifying our water. Normally CO2 is a waste of combustion that our body rejects by pulmonary expiration, so what nonsense it is to swallow so much of it while smoking or drinking sodas. This CO2 is perhaps, moreover, the most harmful element of carbonated drinks, before the added sugar...

The following chapters deal with diabetes, hypertension, cholesterol, obesity, sedentary lifestyle, pollution and chronic problems, conventional treatments to prevent infarction. We learn a lot of details about the toxic drugs and devices used.

The following explains how to change your lifestyle, regarding physical and sexual exercise, stress management, and reviews some alternative medicines, and from page 241, it explains in detail the nutrition to adopt to prevent CVD, and therefore cancer and many other diseases.

It is therefore a very complete, serious and very useful book that I advise to read, or at least to use to change your lifestyle, and therefore be much less sick in the future.□

D / CVD according to Dr. Greger

According to the book by Dr. Michael Greger and his team of volunteer doctors, "Eating better can save your life", from 2018, ISBN 978-2266285155 - (old title: "How not to die?")

It is on page 51 that he tackles the subject: How not to die from a heart disease.

He explains that the fatty deposits that form the atheroma plaque on the inner wall of our arteries are the number one cause of human death. This process builds up over the decades, slowly invading the interior volume of the arteries, blocking the flow of blood, which can cause chest pain when the heart is not getting enough oxygen, known as angina pectoris.

And if a piece of plaque breaks, a blood clot can form in the artery and block it, causing what is called a heart attack, myocardial infarction, which can destroy the heart muscle. It can kill you within an hour.

The general tendency is to consider this as normal wear and tear of the heart, after billions of beats over decades. But large amounts of evidence show that there are places in the world where humans do not suffer from these problems. As in the so-called "Campbell" survey, or "The China Study", which concerns the study of the eating habits of hundreds of thousands of Chinese in rural areas. For example, in the Guizhou region, which includes half a million people, over 3 years, not a single death among those under 65 has been attributed to a coronary problem.

Another example concerns the 1930s and 1940s, and Western missionary doctors who worked in hospitals in sub-Saharan Africa, who noticed that locals did not suffer from the typical deadly diseases that were already devastating more developed countries. In Uganda, a country of several million people, cardiovascular disease was considered almost non-existent. [3]

They carried out autopsies on locals and on Americans of Missouri, of identical ages, and on 632 people on each side, they found 132 deaths by heart attack in the USA, against 1 in Uganda! Ugandans had 100 times fewer heart attacks than Americans in the 1930s.

Shocked by these results, they conducted hundreds of additional autopsies in Uganda, and found only one heart that was slightly damaged, but which had healed, out of a total of 1,400 people. It is not genetic, because studies show that after having emigrated to developed countries, these populations very quickly develop the same diseases when they adopt the modern diet.

Although the diets of these two countries with very low rates of heart disease, China and Uganda, are very different, they have in common that they are based on plants, such as whole grains and vegetables. The high fiber content and the few animal products seem to make the difference.

Coronary artery disease begins in childhood
In 1953, autopsies of 300 Americans who died in the Korean War, showed that 77% of soldiers, aged 22 on average, already had signs of atherosclerosis. Some of these young people even had arteries blocked at 90% or more. [20]

Later it was discovered that the first signs were present in almost all autopsied children over 10 years of age. Complete plaques can appear from the age of 20, and at 40 or 50 they begin to kill us.

More so, doctors have found that the problems begin in the mother's womb, if the mother has high cholesterol levels, the fetus suffers. [23] These days many women quit smoking and drinking while pregnant, but they should also eat better.

Autopsies show that the quantity of plaques is directly linked to the bad LDL cholesterol level in the blood. Dietary cholesterol comes from animal products. The optimal cholesterol level is between 50 and 70 mg / dl, which is the rate present at birth and in populations largely spared from cardiovascular disease, and this would be the rate at which atherosclerosis stops progressing.

The Framingham study reported that no death from coronary artery disease occurs in people with an LDL level of 70 mg / dl, for a total cholesterol of 150 mg / dl. [30]

Dr. Roberts found that there are only 2 ways to achieve 70 mg / dl, either prescribe lifelong treatment for all Americans, or adopt a diet based on whole plant foods. [31]

People do not realize that the drug solution, for example taking statins, is not as effective as intended, and above all it only treats the symptom. On the other hand, it is very lucrative, just the statin of the Lipitor brand brings in 140 billion. [32] Some have even proposed adding it to public drinking water, along with fluorine.

Statins often have other side effects, such as muscle loss, brain damage and memory loss, increased risk of diabetes, and doubling the risk of breast cancer. Why take all these risks, when a plant-based diet has shown that it can lower cholesterol without the risks. [39]

It is even the opposite in terms of side effects, which are positive with the vegetarian diet, with a lower risk of cancer, diabetes and protection of the liver and the brain, as is shown here.

Another chapter is called: Heart disease is reversible.

It's never too late to start eating right, as Nathan Pritikin, Dean Ornish and Caldwell Esselstyn Jr have shown, by taking advanced heart patients, and putting them on the same diet as the Asian and African populations who do not suffer from it. Not only has heart disease stopped progressing, it has reversed! The atheroma plaques gradually dissolved, and the arteries therefore cleared, without surgery, and even in the case where the 3 arteries were affected. The body was only waiting for a healthy diet to repair itself and get back to functioning properly. [40]

This is the well-kept secret of medicine, the body can heal itself, like when you bump or cut yourself. Unless you do it repeatedly on the same place of course, as is the case with poor nutrition. [41]

Endotoxins that damage your arteries

Arteries are not simple mechanical pipes, they are living and dynamic organs. A single fast-food meal can stiffen them in a few hours, reducing their flexibility in half. And it's been known for 20 years. [43]

It is an inflammatory state that lasts for several hours, and when we eat a harmful meal every few hours, we end up putting the body in chronic inflammation mode. The damage of junk food does not happen only after a few decades, but immediately after a bad meal.

For a long time researchers thought that the inflammatory reaction was due to fats or animal proteins, but they recently discovered that they were bacterial toxins, endotoxins. These bacteria that cause inflammation, even when they are dead, are present even in cooked meat. Nothing destroys these toxins. So after a meal with animal products, these toxins can pass into the blood and cause an inflammatory reaction in the arteries, which lasts several hours. [44]

Dr. Ornish reported 91% less chest pain in patients who had been eating mostly vegetarian for only a few weeks. The body repairs itself very quickly, with or without physical exercise. [45, 46] Of course, the complete cleaning of the atheroma plaques takes longer. By comparison, those who just followed the prescriptions of their doctor, experienced in the same period, an increase of 186% in attacks of angina pectoris! [47]

References:
[3] 1959 https://www.ncbi.nlm.nih.gov/pubmed/23045195
[20] 1960 https://www.ncbi.nlm.nih.gov/pubmed/13838030
[23] 1997 https://www.ncbi.nlm.nih.gov/pubmed/9389731
[30=31] 2008 https://www.ncbi.nlm.nih.gov/pubmed/18849550
[39] 2003 https: //www .ncbi.nlm.nih.gov / pubmed / 14527636
[40] 2010 https://www.ncbi.nlm.nih.gov/pubmed/20816134
[41] 2012 https://www.ncbi.nlm.nih.gov / pubmed / 22561031
[43] 1997 https://www.ncbi.nlm.nih.gov/pubmed/9036757
[44] 2011 https://www.ncbi.nlm.nih.gov/pubmed/20849668
[45=47] 1998 https://www.ncbi.nlm.nih.gov/pubmed/9863851
[46] 1983 https://www.ncbi.nlm.nih.gov/pubmed/6336794

2. Preventing Cancers

All cancers are the second leading cause of death worldwide.

A / "Official speech" summarizes what the medical authorities say.

B / "Niedzwiecki and Rath Theory" presents the book by Doctors Niedzwiecki and Rath which deals with cancer. The seriousness of the speakers and the theory should prompt us to try it on a large-scale scientific study, since it would cure cancer in any situation, regardless of a change in diet and lifestyle.

C / "Lyon Study" presents extracts from the book by Doctor de Lorgeril, who was the main investigator of the famous "Lyon Study" which scientifically proved the remarkable effectiveness of a change in lifestyle and adoption of a traditional Mediterranean type diet, against CVD, but also against cancer.

D / "Anti-cancer" concerns the book by Doctor Greger, who with his team of volunteer doctors, reviews hundreds of scientific publications every week.

E / "Dr. Schwartz" presents the theory and the supplements discovered by Doctor Schwartz which block the development of cancer.

F / "Pr Beljanski" quickly presents the discovery of this doctor who also cured cancers with supplements.

G / "Bicarbonate" presents the theory of Doctor Simoncini who destroys many tumors with his very simple method.

H / "Vitamin C" presents some information from different Doctors who have used ascorbic acid against cancer.

A / Cancer, the official speech

According to the World Health Organization

According to its official website in French:
https://www.who.int/topics/cancer/fr/

Cancer is a general term applied to a large group of diseases that can affect any part of the body. One of its characteristics is the rapid proliferation of abnormal cells which can swarm in other organs, forming what are called metastases. Many cancers can be prevented by avoiding the main risk factors, such as smoking. A significant number of cancers can be treated with surgery, radiotherapy and chemotherapy, especially if they are detected early enough.

Cancer prevention

At least a third of all cancer cases are preventable. Prevention is the most cost-effective long-term strategy for fighting cancer.

Smoking is the single largest preventable risk factor for cancer mortality worldwide as it causes an estimated 22% of cancer deaths per year. In 2004, 1.6 million of the 7.4 million cancer deaths were due to smoking.

Sedentary lifestyle, dietary factors, obesity and overweight

Changing your eating habits is another important way to fight cancer. There is a link between overweight / obesity and many types of cancer such as esophagus, colon and rectum, breast, endometrium and kidney. Diets rich in fruits and vegetables could have a protective effect against many cancers. Conversely, excessive consumption of red or canned meat may be associated with an increased risk of colorectal cancer. In addition, healthy eating habits that prevent the onset of diet-related cancers will also lower the risk of cardiovascular disease.

Regular physical exercise and maintaining a normal body weight, combined with a healthy diet, will greatly reduce the risk of cancer. National policies and programs need to be implemented to raise awareness and reduce exposure to cancer risk factors, and to ensure that they receive the information and support they need to adopt healthy living habits. healthy lives.

Alcohol consumption

Alcohol consumption is a risk factor for many types of cancer, including those of the oral cavity, pharynx, larynx, esophagus, liver, colon, rectum and breast. The risk of cancer increases with the amount of alcohol consumed.

Environmental

Air pollution, water and soil pollution by carcinogenic chemicals explains 1% to 4% of all cancers (IARC / WHO, 2003).

Occupational

More than 40 carcinogens agents, mixtures and modes of exposure present in the professional environment are carcinogenic for humans and therefore classified as occupational carcinogens (Siemiatycki et al., 2004).

Cancer according to the American Institute for Cancer Research
According to their official website: https://www.aicr.org
The ten recommendations for cancer prevention:
Maintaining a healthy weight is the most important thing you can do to reduce your risk of cancer.
Physical activity in all its forms helps reduce the risk of cancer.
Basing our diets on plant foods (such as vegetables, fruits, whole grains and beans), which contain fiber and other nutrients, can reduce our risk of cancer.
There is strong evidence that the consumption of "fast foods" and a "Western-style" diet are causes of weight gain, overweight and obesity, linked to 12 cancers.
The expert group recommends limiting red meat and avoiding processed meat.
There is strong evidence that the consumption of sugary drinks leads to weight gain, overweight and obesity, linked to 12 cancers.
For cancer prevention, the evidence is clear and convincing: alcohol, whatever its form, is a potent carcinogen.
Caution against waiting for any dietary supplement to reduce the risk of cancer as much as a healthy diet can do.
According to the expert report, breastfeeding benefits both the mother and the child.
Anyone who has been diagnosed with cancer should receive specialized nutritional advice from a trained professional.

Cancer according to Dr. Axel Kahn, President of the French National League Against Cancer.
According to an interview published in the magazine "Pour la science Hors-Série" n 105 of December 2019.
In this interview he explains that he was working on the adaptation and regulation of liver genes in relation to food. They had identified several mechanisms that explain how glucose influences gene expression. And in 2002 came the first studies linking the state of children's health to the amount of food available for their grandparents. They discovered a form of non-genetic inheritance.
He says that yes, genes act according to the code they contain, but they are also controlled, in the short and long term, by all the epigenetic mechanisms, which are the manifestation of the environment.
To the question, does epigenetics intervene in the formation of cancers, he replies, I quote:
"To my knowledge, changes in the level of expression of genes alone are incapable of causing cancer. Special conditions need to exist (ionizing radiation, pollution, inflammation, etc.)"

And lo and behold, pollutant toxins and inflammation trigger cancer, not just gene mutations or changes in their expression!

Second major problem, the fact that cancer cells become invisible to the immune system, which does not attack them. Because I quote: "the cancer cell is capable of inactivating the immune cells so as not to be destroyed".

Therefore, any anticancer action will have to come from outside our body, since our defense system no longer works. Many studies on the micronutrients present in fruits and vegetables in particular, show their blocking effects on the development of cancers.

Later in this interview, concerning the role of inflammation and the microbiota, Professor Kahn recalls that the main risk factors for cancer, by number of deaths in France, are tobacco (45,000 deaths), alcohol (15,000) and obesity (3,500).

Their next campaign will focus on junk food and obesity... why not focus on good food and the joy of being active? Indeed, it is a joy to eat fresh fruits and vegetables, as well as to exercise physically. And these two habits solve, as if by chance, most health problems.

He adds that the inflammation is the first factor of carcinogenesis, then it is the modification of the metabolism, and finally the intestinal microbiota...

Here, by dint of beating around the bush for decades, they will end up falling into it; Yes, indeed, citizens, it is our diet and our physical activity that largely determine our good health.□

B / Cancer by Drs Rath and Niedzwiecki

According to the book by Dr Matthias Rath and Aleksandra Niedzwiecki, "Victory over cancer - Cancer, the end of a disease of civilization - Book I - The scientific breakthrough", from 2011, ISBN 978-9076332826. Free on their official website: http://www.dr-rath-foundation.org/2018/08/victory-over-cancer/

Selected extracts: "This book documents a revolutionary scientific discovery that will lead to natural cancer control, without having to develop new high-tech research.

It is no coincidence that the role of micronutrients in the fight against cancer is neither understood nor applied in the fight against this disease. It was deliberately set aside and kept for the benefit of the pharmaceutical industry and its profits.

This book gives millions of people the opportunity to act and end dependence on health for economic interests."

"For millennia, a disease which, until today, was largely incurable has struck humanity: it is cancer. For nearly a century, this disease has been the target of an investment industry, the pharmaceutical sector, which has made the multi-billion dollar business of the cancer epidemic. The result was predictable. At the start of the 21st century, this disease continues to spread worldwide; for most types of cancer, the annual death toll is continuously increasing and health care costs attributable to chemotherapy and other questionable methods of care are exploding and financially ruining both patients and the community."

This book ends this tragedy. The natural healing methods presented in this book are able - which has been scientifically proven - to inhibit all of the key mechanisms in cancer cells that make cancer a deadly disease.

The Facts

Fact # 1: In 2008, in North America and Europe alone, 5.6 million people die from cancer each year. In 2010, chemotherapy sessions alone cost the US $ 56 billion.

Fact # 2: The cancer epidemic continues to spread, despite all the hype that is made about so-called "breakthroughs" in the fight against this disease.

Fact # 3: The therapeutic goal of chemotherapy and radiation therapy is to kill cancer cells by intoxicating the entire body.

Fact # 4: The toxicity of chemotherapy is frightening. Chemotherapy owes its origin to the molecules of mustard gas from the 1st World War.

Fact # 5: Toxic substances used in chemotherapy lead to increased consumption of other drugs.

Key mechanisms

The production of enzymes which degrade collagen is the essential condition for the development of cancer and its spread, whatever its form and whatever organ in which the primary tumor has grown. And all cancer cells use enzymes that destroy collagen to form metastases in other organs. With the publication of this book, the mechanisms of metastasis formation are "demystified" and now understandable by everyone.

Lysine as an essential agent

Two groups of molecules are capable of blocking these mechanisms of degradation of collagen. The first group is that of endogenous enzyme inhibitors which can stop in a few moments the action of those which destroy collagen. The second group consists of components of our diet or food supplements that block enzymes.

The most important of these substances is the natural amino acid L-lysine. A sufficiently large quantity of lysine brought in through food or food supplements makes it possible to block the anchor points used by the enzymes for the degradation of collagen to attach to the molecules of the connective tissue. Lysine can in this way inhibit uncontrolled breakdown of connective tissue. Our body can store large amounts of lysine and the daily intake of several grams of this amino acid has no side effects, because it knows this molecule and it simply excretes the unused amounts.

How much lysine can our body absorb?

- A human body weighing 75 kg contains about 11 kg of protein.
- 50% of this mass are proteins from connective tissue, collagen and elastin.
- The amino acid lysine constitutes approximately 12% of the mass of collagen and elastin.
- A human body weighing 75 kg therefore contains approximately 500 gr of lysine.

Healthy collagen: The key to disease prevention and control is optimal production of collagen molecules that are essential for healthy connective tissue and that form the basis for effective control of cancer and other diseases.

Vitamin C: Catalyzes and controls the production of collagen in the nucleus of cells. Vitamin C also stimulates the formation of chemical "bridges" between the collagen fibers, which gives good stability to the entire structure.

Lysine: Constituent element of collagen, brought only through food. Our body cannot produce lysine on its own.

Proline: Another important building block amino acid in collagen. Proline can be synthesized by our body, but only in limited quantities. If a person has a chronic disease (causing long-term enzymatic breakdown of collagen), the body's ability to produce proline may be depleted.

Why is it not recognized?

Currently, several thousand cancer patients have sent us testimonials, and many have attached copies of their medical records. More than 10 years after being diagnosed with cancer, many people are leading normal lives today.

Chapter 3 deals with the scientific facts that make this breakthrough irreversible, by Dr. Niedzwiecki. In 1999, when they created their own Research Institute, Dr. Rath asked her to take charge of it. Thanks to pioneers in cancer research, such as Dr. Shrirang Netke and, subsequently, Dr. Waheed Roomi, their work in this area has been able to progress very quickly. As early as 2001, they knew that the direction given by Dr. Rath's concept, developed ten years earlier, was the right one. Their first challenge was to identify the most effective group of natural substances that would slow the spread of cancer cells in the body. To date, they have published more than 60 scientific reports on this subject. They are going to tell you many facts about the incredible possibility of finally being able to beat cancer.

In addition to vitamin C and lysine, there are certain other important micronutrients that can help naturally block the mechanisms of this disease; and all these micronutrients together have a synergistic effect, i.e. that they play a team role and thus mutually reinforce their effect in cancer control.

The key mechanisms of cancer
Diffusion of cancer cells and formation of metastases
Multiplication of cancer cells and development of tumor
Formation of new tumor blood vessels (angiogenesis)
Triggering of the natural death of cancer cells (apoptosis)
Micronutrients important for naturally controlling cancer

This micronutrient "team" can be broken down into several groups according to certain mechanisms of action that are important in controlling cancer. These include, for example:

• supporting the production of connective tissue and maintaining its stability: vitamin C, lysine, proline, copper, manganese.

• inhibitors of the breakdown of connective tissue: lysine, proline, vitamin C, N-acetylcysteine (NAC), green tea, selenium.

• inhibitors of the formation of new blood vessels (angiogenesis): green tea, NAC.

• factors triggering the death of cancer cells (apoptosis): vitamin C, green tea, NAC, selenium, arginine, proline.

The higher the concentration of micronutrients, the more the degradation of the surrounding collagen is reduced.

Micronutrients prevent the spread of more than 40 types of human cancer

We tested the synergistic effect of these micronutrients on more than 40 different types of human cancer. Among the types of cancer studied are some of the forms that most commonly affect millions of people, such as cancer of the lungs, colon, pancreas, skin, ovaries, blood and many more.

The results of our work on this large number of human cancers have shown us that the combination of micronutrients studied makes it possible to completely stop the spread of all the cancer cell lines that we have tested. The only difference was the concentration of micronutrients needed to reach this goal.

Of course, this does not mean that micronutrients can stop the progression of cancer, regardless of its stage. This is especially true when the disease is at an advanced stage, as well as when the immune system - and therefore the body's ability to fight the disease - has been destroyed by "chemotherapy".

Complete inhibition with low micronutrient concentration:
- Breast cancer - Hodgkin's lymphoma Complete inhibition with moderate micronutrient concentration - Lung cancer - Colon cancer - Cervical cancer - Skin cancer (melanoma) - Bone cancer (osteosarcoma) - Testicular cancer - Blood cancer (non-Hodgkin's lymphoma) - Pancreatic cancer.

Complete inhibition with a high concentration of micronutrients:
- Liver cancer - Bladder cancer - Kidney cancer - Ovarian cancer - Prostate cancer - Brain tumor (glioblastoma) - Blood cancer (leukemia, LMP)

Our Research Institute is not influenced by pharmaceutical investment activities, nor by any other private financial investor. Our Research Institute and the entire Dr Rath group of companies belong to a non-profit foundation. Therefore, we do not profit by sharing this information with you. Our only interest is your health. Is there a better way to gain your trust?

Website www.drrathresearch.org. Official website of our California Research Institute http://www.wha-www.org/en/library/index.html

The second volume of their book is also available for free download, "Cancer The end of a disease of civilization - Book II - Investment trade with cancer is going to end ", ISBN 9076332835.

Book II - Investment trade with cancer is going to end.
Throughout its history, humanity has constantly been condemned to relive the worst tragedies it had ever known, for a very simple reason: the generation that came after each of these disasters had forgotten the lessons of the past. The cancer epidemic, which alone claimed the lives of more than a billion people in the 20th century, is no exception. The scientific breakthrough documented in Book I provides the scientific basis for the end of the "cancer epidemic". However, the end of this disease of civilization that is cancer will only be possible if: - we provide an answer to the question of knowing for what reasons this breakthrough is only happening now, - we are openly citing economic forces , whose existence depends largely on the persistence of the cancer epidemic, - we bring to light the dark past of these interest groups, - we learn from history. This book is the basic document which will allow humanity to assert its right to live in a "world without cancer". □

C / Cancer according to Dr. de Lorgeril

According to the books by Dr. de Lorgeril, "The new Mediterranean diet. To protect your health and the planet", from 2017, ISBN 978-2501111898, and "Preventing a heart attack and stroke", from 2011, ISBN 978-2916878881

In terms of food, the modernized Mediterranean diet is most effective in preventing cancer, according to scientific results. The Mediterranean diet is undoubtedly an anticancer diet. Be careful, good eating habits must be kept all the time. Cancer that begins at retirement age has taken decades to form, and therefore started as early as 30 years of age, for example. The average age of a person who dies of cancer is 60 years.

The Lyon Heart study on the Mediterranean diet initiated by Dr de Lorgeril is the international benchmark on the subject, and after such spectacular results more than 20 years ago, it is obvious that the authorities in place do not want to discover all the positive effects of a suitable diet, since no follow-up was given. Perhaps one day our societies will change, and their citizens will finally experience good health without pills, knowing what is good or not to eat.

He explains the Warburg effect of glucose fermentation by cancer cells (cancer theory adopted by Dr. Laurent Schwartz who recommends a ketogenic diet in some cases), and says that it is a good idea to adopt an anti-diabetic diet or at least poor in sugars, with a low glycemic index, which will reduce the peaks of glucose and insulin in the blood.

He also presents another theory: muscle cells in the arterial wall that migrate and proliferate. Biologists developed this theory in the 1970s. Atherosclerotic plaques are thought to be due to a tumor proliferation of muscle cells, taking the form of plaques. This is how they discovered the first tumor growth factor, PDGF (Platelet-derived growth factor).

It all started from the observation that people at high risk of cancer are also at high risk of cardiovascular disease. All these diseases are caused by our new way of life! After some angioplasty procedures on arteries we can sometimes quickly see the proliferation of plaques by cell migration and their tumoral multiplication that can go up to clogging the artery.

Most of the eating habits of traditional Mediterranean are:
Vegetables are the basis of the meal
They consume animal products in a moderate way
They take advantage of a very wide dietary diversity
They eat according to the seasons
They eat a lot of whole grains, vegetables and dried fruits and vegetables.

He explains that it was Ancel Keys, in the USA after the Second World War, who spoke of the "Mediterranean diet", after having found that the Mediterranean populations were free from coronary artery disease, when it was already the first cause of mortality in the USA.

And it was Serge Renaud who revived the concept in the 1980s, speaking of the "Cretan regime", based on "the study of the 7 countries" by Keys. [1] It was at the famous INSERM unit 63 in Lyon, France, from where Michel de Lorgeril will launch the "Lyon study" aimed at testing the effectiveness of this regime on patients already victims of a heart attack. [2]

This study found fewer cardiac deaths and myocardial infarction, 50 to 70% less risk, and less other complications, less pulmonary embolism, less stroke, less heart failure, but also fewer cancers, and an improvement in life expectancy.

This greatly surprised all the scientists taking part in the study. So, they decided to check everything out, and find no errors or biases. It was one of the most meticulously researched study, having given such unexpected results to doctors and scientists who considered food to be unrelated to good health.

The range of health effects from the traditional Mediterranean diet is vast. It protects against cardiovascular diseases of all types, and therefore also against high blood pressure, but also against diabetes, gout, and of course against cancers and inflammatory diseases, as well as against overweight and obesity, and against metabolic syndromes (pre-diabetes).

The key foods are, in summary, vegetables and legumes in quantity but also of great variety, seasonal fruits, including citrus fruits present in the Mediterranean, whole grains, and especially rustic wheat low in gluten.

The fat comes mainly from olive and rapeseed oils, then from seafood, which also provides high quality protein, iodine, B12, minerals and omega-3 much needed and beneficial.

And finally, farm products, especially poultry and rabbits, eggs and fermented dairy products, such as yogurts and sheep and goat cheese. Cows are rarely present on the Mediterranean coasts. Meat is considered a condiment and not the basis of the meal, unlike what we do now, while in addition we have become very sedentary. Cold meats are only present in certain areas.

In the Lyon study, the average was 30% lipids, including 8% saturated fat. Cooking is done in a simple way, with little or no cooking, and at low temperature, with rare fried foods. He specifies that this Mediterranean model can be modified by removing one of the elements, such as alcohol for anti alcohol, or wheat bread for anti gluten. Even if these foods have special advantages that can almost be considered protective. And he recalls the importance of our intestinal bacteria which participate in our metabolism.

Lifestyle is crucial

He tells 3 stories that led him to these nutritional choices to prevent diseases, including cardiovascular or cancer. This book is not a new anti-cancer diet, but it turns out that these lifestyle changes are also protective against this disease. There is no set number of protective factors, but it is a lifestyle package that needs to be adopted.

He says that it is the same scientific logic as against CVD, since it was during this very supervised study in Lyon that he discovered in 1998 that this Mediterranean diet also protects very significantly against cancer.

Anti-cancer diets

This is a complicated subject, but the general principle is to try to help the immune system or the therapies undertaken, such as chemotherapy, radiotherapy or surgery, while protecting healthy cells as much as possible. Our existence necessarily leads to the creation of cancer cells, which our system must eliminate, and we must do our best to help it and prevent their progression into tumors. We must therefore fight against the degradation of our DNA, thanks to the antioxidants in our diet.

He talks about suppressing oxygen, which is also necessary for tumor cells, which seems difficult, because without oxygen we die! In any case, physical exercise is recognized as helping to prevent cancer, which paradoxically strongly oxygenates the body. But he explains that it could be the brevity of the oxidative stress generated by physical exertion, which would stimulate the immune system. Maybe too much sport would become counterproductive?

Anti-cholesterol drugs

Regarding diabetes and cancer, they have had parallel progress in our societies. So a success against cancer will go through a success against diabetes and pre-diabetes. The same goes for prevention, one goes with the other. He says that it is absurd to prescribe cholesterol-lowering drugs (including statins), which are useless for preventing cardiovascular disease, but which in addition increase the risk of diabetes in a tragic way, up to 60% in postmenopausal women, who are most at risk of developing cancer. Statins can do a lot of harm, and also increase the risk of depression and the risk of cancer.

Breast or ovarian cancers are much more common in carriers of the BRCA1 or 2 gene, although some never suffer from it. Hormone treatments for menopause have been found to increase the number of cancers and cardiovascular disease. Today women smoke more than men, and we see an increase in bronchial cancer and cardiovascular disease in this population.

Sedentary lifestyle

Physical exercise protects us from cardiovascular disease, hypertension, diabetes and pre-diabetes, obesity, and even cancer. We have solid scientific data showing that physical exercise is more effective than drugs in reducing overweight, diabetes and also cancers and cardiovascular diseases.

Alcohol and cancer

He says that it all depends on the dose, and that without excess it is not a problem. He does not share the opinion of the National Cancer Institute (INCa) on this subject. But there would be an exception for breast cancer, since each glass of alcohol would increase the risk by 10%. So even a low consumption would be dangerous in this case, except, according to studies, if the woman is a large consumer of plants containing group B vitamins. Only the Mediterranean diet would be protective for women, and they could continue to drink wine while eating. Teas are also very rich in polyphenols, especially green tea, some of which could reduce the risk of prostate cancer.

There are unfortunately only 2 pages on vitamin C, and 10 studies cited, all using very small doses compared to the recommendations by doctors who have had success with it, and 2 relate to plants. Collagen is mentioned but not in the measure of its proven critical role for the human body.

The Lyon study did not study this cancer regime, but all cases were recorded and documented during the 4 years of follow-up. There was less cancer in the group with the least omega-6, these being pro-inflammatory. It was the Lyon study that launched the anti-cancer nutrition movement. More than a dozen groups then conducted epidemiological studies on various populations around the world, and confirmed the results of the Lyon study, i.e. fewer cancers and better life expectancy. It is the only dietary model that has been proven scientifically.

He deplores the fact that all of this remained hidden, particularly in France, until the publication in 2007 of the book "Anticancer" by David Servan-Schreiber", that is to say 10 years after the publication of the results of the Lyon Study against cancer.

It is time for doctors to realize that modern imaging and detection techniques are useless for prevention, since they can only work when the disease is already in place.

[1] 1984 https://www.ncbi.nlm.nih.gov/pubmed/6739443 PMID: 6739443
The study of the seven countries: 2,289 deaths in 15 years.

[2] 1994-1999 INSERM, Etude de Lyon
1994 https://www.ncbi.nlm.nih.gov/pubmed/7911176?dopt=Abstract
Mediterranean diet rich in alpha-linolenic acid in secondary disease prevention coronary.
1999 https://www.ncbi.nlm.nih.gov/pubmed/9989963?dopt=Abstract
Mediterranean diet, traditional risk factors and rate of cardiovascular complications after myocardial infarction: final report of the Lyon Diet study Heart.

The lyon study (by Inserm at Bron) in 1994, the most serious ever, had found a reduction of 73% in deaths from cardiovascular disease and myocardial infarction, after a dietary change by adoption of a Mediterranean diet!
The results 5 years later were confirmed:
"Conclusions of 1999: The protective effect of the Mediterranean diet was maintained until 4 years after the first heart attack, confirming the previous intermediate analyzes. The main traditional risk factors, such as high cholesterol and high blood pressure, have proven to be independent and joint predictors of recidivism, indicating that the Mediterranean diet has not changed, at least qualitatively, the usual relationships between the main risk factors and recurrence. Thus, an overall strategy to reduce cardiovascular morbidity and mortality should mainly include a cardioprotective diet. It should be combined with other (pharmacological?) means aimed at reducing modifiable risk factors. Other trials combining the two approaches are warranted."□

D / Cancer according to Dr. Greger

According to the book by Dr. Michael Greger and his team of volunteer Doctors, "Eating better can save your life", 2018, ISBN 978-2266285155 - (old title: "How not to die?")

A healthy diet can protect DNA damage and even prevent cancer. Lung cancer is the worst death he has ever seen. It is the deadliest, yet it could be avoided, and kills 160,000 people a year, a direct result of smoking. It is diagnosed 200,000 times per year in the USA, more than the following 3 forms of cancer, colon, breast and pancreas combined. [1]

Heart disease is not yet recognized as the consequence of poor diet; however it is recognized that 90% of lung cancer is caused by tobacco. Male smokers are 23 times more likely to develop one, and female smokers 13 times more, compared to non-smokers. The tobacco industry has always hired doctors to advertise cigarettes. Then in the 1980s, they hired doctors and scientists to produce studies that denied the tobacco and cancer relationship. No wonder so many people have started smoking, and habits are so hard to change. [4]

Stop immediately, and only 20 minutes later your heart will calm down and your blood pressure will drop, and within a few weeks your blood circulation and lung function will improve. In a few months, the eyelashes used to clean the pulmonary alveoli will grow back, and before 1 year without smoking, your risk of coronary heart disease will have decreased by 50%. [5] Our body has an incredible capacity for regeneration, give it this chance. 85% of women with lung cancer die within 5 years, 90% from metastasis, the spread of cancer. [8]

Smoked Food

A quarter of lung cancers affect people who have never smoked. [21] Part of it is due to passive smoking, but cooking food, especially frying, releases carcinogenic toxins, even before the appearance of smoke. [22,23,24] So think of adding good ventilation in your kitchen. Some foods like meat and fish seem to be more carcinogenic than others, bacon being the worst. [25,32]

Stock up on broccoli

The smoke itself contains many toxins that weaken the immune system, and they can even damage DNA. [6] Scientists have studied the protective power of broccoli in smokers. With one serving a day, after 10 days, DNA damage had decreased by 41%. This is proof that vegetables have powerful protective effects, even for our DNA. [7]

How not to die from digestive cancer

Colorectal cancer kills 50 thousand Americans each year, 40 thousand for the pancreas, and 18 thousand for the esophagus cancer.

Anti-cancer protective agents can be classified into different categories:

- those that prevent the development of cancer
- the antioxidants that prevent DNA mutation
- and those that prevent the proliferation and growth of tumors

Curcumin is special because it acts in these three areas. For example, 38% less DNA mutation with 1 teaspoon per day of commercial turmeric powder. [13,14,15,16]

The cancer rate is much lower in India than in the USA. Americans have 10 times more colorectal cancers than Indians, 17 times more lung cancers, 12 times more kidney cancers, 8 times more bladder cancers, and 5 times more breast cancers!

It's about the same ratios for men elsewhere.

The use of turmeric in the daily diet has been put forward as a reason for this. By studying smokers, they found that by eating turmeric, cancerous structures in the rectum decreased by 40%. And the only negative effect was the staining of yellow stool. [16] And for already installed cancerous polyps, a reduction of 50% after 6 months, if we add quercetin to curcumin (found in red onions and grapes). [17] And when colorectal cancer is already developed and intractable by chemotherapy or radiation, within a few months, turmeric extract has interrupted the progression of cancer in 33% of patients. [18]

Despite these impressive life-saving rates, superior to chemo and radiation, turmeric is never proposed as the first treatment for cancer... it is certain that without a patentable element, there is no financial point to this, and yet so much life and suffering would be spared. [19]

The very low cancer rates in India can be explained by the spices they use daily, but also by the fact that they are the biggest consumers of fruits and vegetables, and only 7% of the population adult consumes meat daily. [20] They consume green vegetables every day, legumes such as beans, split peas, chickpeas and lentils, very rich in anti-cancer agents.

Phytates

The key against colorectal cancer seems to be fibers. In Uganda, which had the lowest rate recorded, surgeon Denis Burkitt spent 24 years working there in different hospitals, never having had to treat a single case of colon cancer. After all this research he concluded that it was the amount of fiber that made the difference, Ugandans mainly eating whole plant foods. [30,31,32,33]

But globally, research has shown that it does not depend on the amount of fiber ingested, but perhaps phytates, present in the seeds of plants, therefore in whole grains, beans, nuts and seeds. [34,35,36] Phytates remove excess iron from the body, thus avoiding the generation of harmful free radicals. [36] Meat contains a type of iron that is very associated with colon cancer, which would make it doubly harmful. [37]

Please note that refined, incomplete whole plant foods do not contain phytates. Phytates have recently been shown to facilitate the absorption of minerals, it was previously thought to be the opposite, and therefore people who consume the most phytate-rich foods have better bone density and less hip fracture. They act like anti osteoporosis drugs, but without the sometimes catastrophic side effects.[41,42,43,44]

Phytates inhibit the growth of almost all cancer cells, colon, breast, uterus, prostate, liver, pancreas and skin. [48,49] They also enhance the action of white blood cells. [51] And they can interrupt the feeding of existing tumors. [52]

8 times less risk of colon cancer with a diet rich in plant products and low in meat. [46] A simple change can already do a lot. The US National Cancer Institute has found that adding 50 grams of beans a day reduces the recurrence of colorectal polyps by 65%. [47]

Pancreatic cancer

It is the most fatal of all, only 6% of patients survive after 5 years. 20% could be caused by smoking, then obesity and alcohol consumption.

Chicken and pancreatic cancer

The EPIC study, on 477,000 individuals, concluded that there was a 72% increase in the risk of pancreatic cancer for those who ate 50 grams of chicken per day. It is the equivalent of a small piece of chicken breast. [90]

In the laboratory, curcumin has shown effects against cancer cells in the pancreas. [95] But some tumors may be resistant to curcumin, only 2% of tumors reacted positively to curcumin, but this is equivalent to the results of chemo. For this dazzling cancer, prevention is the vital condition, and therefore requires a healthy diet, no tobacco, alcohol or obesity.

Esophageal cancer

18,000 new cases in the USA and 15,000 deaths. Main risk from smoking; then the gastric reflux which creates an inflammation of the walls, which can be changed by food. Alcohol increasing the risk.

Blood cancers, leukemias

These are tumors that circulate in the blood instead of accumulating in one place. They often start in the bone marrow, where red and white blood cells and platelets are made. At Oxford University, they followed 60,000 people and found that vegetarians have less risk of cancer, and half the risk of developing leukemia than those who eat meat. [6,7]

Certain molecules present in vegetables can act. Sulforaphane, contained in cruciferous plants (broccoli, cauliflower, kale, other cabbage, turnips, arugula, radish, etc.) kills leukemia cells in the laboratory. [8] In a study of 500 women with leukemia, undergoing chemo and radiation treatment, those eating 3 servings of vegetables per week had a 40% higher survival rate. [9] The Iowa study of 35,000 women also concluded that those who ate vegetables were less at risk. [11] That of the Mayo clinic leads to the same conclusions, with 5 servings of vegetables per week, the risk is halved. [12]

The antioxidants in these vegetables act strongly against cancer, but not antioxidant supplements. For example, in 2010, a large intake of vitamin C through the diet reduced the risk of lymphoma, but a higher dose of vitamin C (300 mg / day) in pill form did not seem beneficial. Same observation with the antioxidant carotenoids. [13,14]

Supplements contain only a few antioxidants, while our cells use hundreds of them in synergy. Fruits and vegetables are the best choice since they contain a huge variety of active molecules.

We can see that Dr. Greger doesn't know or reference to the successes of high doses vitamin C treatments, like mentionned further in this book, with doses in the dozens or hundreds of grams per day.

Breast cancer

Each year 40,000 women die in the USA, and 230,000 are diagnosed.

By the time doctors detect a tumor, it may have been present for 40 years or more. [2] It can take a very long time to develop. Some may even start in the fetus because of the mother's diet and lifestyle. [4,5]

The American Institute for Cancer Research has recommendations that can be summarized as follows: "Diets based on whole foods of plant origin, vegetables, whole grains, fruits and legumes, reduce the risks of many cancers, as well as other diseases". [13]

The follow-up of 30,000 postmenopausal women without a history of breast cancer, showed a fall of 60% of the risks, following only 3 of the 10 recommendations of the Institute, that is to limit alcohol, to eat mainly foods of vegetable origin and maintain a normal weight. The positive effects of a lifestyle change develop from the first weeks of healthy living. The decrease in animal proteins is a major factor, since they contain the cancer growth hormone called IGF-1. [16,17]

Carcinogenic grills

As early as 1939 we discovered the presence of carcinogenic substances in grilled foods. Now identified, these are HA, heterocyclic amines, compounds that are formed when muscle tissue of beef, pork, fish and poultry is cooked at high temperature, in a pan or grill. [51,52]

Cholesterol and cancer

LDL cholesterol stimulates the growth of cancer cells, which feed on it amazingly, and use it for various actions. [76,78,79] But cholesterol-lowering drugs are associated with higher risks of cancer. A study published in 2013 concludes that women who have taken statins for a decade are twice as likely to develop breast cancer. [83]

Prostate cancer and milk

28,000 deaths in the USA each year. Man is the only one to continue drinking milk after his maternal weaning. It contains growth hormones that seem to stimulate the growth of cancer. Many links have been discovered between taking dairy products and cancer, as confirmed by Harvard scientists. [9,10,11]

For example, prostate cancer has multiplied by 25 in Japan since the Second World War, which coincides with a change in their diet, in particular a consumption of eggs multiplied by 7, of meat by 9, and dairy products by 20! [13]

This has also happened in many other countries. [14] Many studies are cited which show the increase in cancers with the regular consumption of dairy products ...

And since it is now established that dairy products do not contribute to bone strength, except during adolescence. There too, the scientific studies cited are numerous. And the results even show negative effects for adult milk drinkers, such as increased fractures, cardiovascular disease, and cancer, for each additional glass of milk, especially for women. 3 glasses of milk per day are associated with a doubling of premature mortality for women and men. [25,26,27,28,31]

Eggs, choline and cancer

A Harvard study that followed 1,000 men with prostate cancer, shows that one egg per day multiplies the progression of said cancer and bone metastases. The only food worse than eggs is poultry. Chicken and turkey eaters quadrupled the risk of spreading cancer. [33]

It is the toxins from cooking that seem to accumulate more in poultry meat than in others. [34] It seems that for eggs, choline is responsible, since a high blood level of choline has been associated with the increase in prostate cancer. [35,36,37,38]

The Harvard team concludes that men who eat 2.5 eggs per week see their risk of dying from prostate cancer increased by 81%! [39] Egg choline, like meat carnitine, is transformed into trimethylamine toxin by the microbiota of carnivores. [40,41] This toxin, once oxidized in the liver, also increases the risks of heart attack, stroke and premature death. [42]

Industrialists know this, but hide it. Fortunately, as Dr. Ornish has demonstrated in his clinical studies, switching to a vegan diet can slow the development of cancer, and even reverse it in some subjects.□

E / Cancer according to Dr. Schwartz

According to the books by Dr. Laurent Schwartz, "The end of diseases?" in 2019, ISBN 979-1020907059, "Cancer: A simple and non-toxic treatment", from 2016, ISBN 978-2365491778, "Cancer - Cure all the sick?" in 2013, ISBN 978-2755611472

And his website: https://guerir-du-cancer.fr/

Doctor Laurent Schwartz (author of the best-seller Cancer: a simple and non-toxic treatment) devoted his life to study cancer and patient care, in France and the United States. Renowned oncologist, trained in Strasbourg and Harvard. Long seconded to the French Ecole Polytechnique, he abandoned the usual oncology practice to look for a more effective way to fight cancer. His research has led him to constitute, within the École Polytechnique, a multidisciplinary laboratory, bringing together doctors, biologists, chemists, mathematicians and physicists.

After years of research on this disease that terrorizes us, Dr. Laurent Schwartz finally presents his conclusions to the public. Prefaced by Professor Luc Montagnier, Nobel Prize in Medicine, he returns to the first encouraging results of his metabolic treatment consisting in positively reprogramming cancer cells rather than systematically destroying them. We don't cure cancer more today than we did 30 years ago, and we die just as much, and we see a global explosion in the number of cancers, and mortality among young people is increasing.

He retained the theory of the Warburg effect, from the Nobel Prize in Medicine Otto Warburg, as a cancer process, it is the fermentation of cells which no longer burn sugar, due to intense inflammation, which ends up causing cancer. He mentioned in one of his lectures that in the past, scientists, to cause cancer in a mouse, rubbed it for a long time to create a strong inflammation, which then turned into cancer.

He tried hundreds of molecules on almost 20,000 mice, to find a synergy of simple molecules that could be effective, because if a single molecule was enough, it would already have been found. He does not seem to know the work of Dr. Matthias Rath with Dr. Aleksandra Niedzwiecki, who took the same path, but sought synergies from more than 2 molecules, adding as long as the results were not satisfactory.

Dr. Schwartz also explains in a 2019 conference at the city of sciences of La Villette, that he does not know anything about vitamin C, but that on the other hand he knew a patient whose file he was able to verify, who was cured with massive injections of vitamin C. (https://youtu.be/5_6_z_DPwxY)

He explains that the cell's cytoplasm is rich in potassium and low in sodium, and the nerve impulse is propagated by an incoming flow of sodium and leaving potassium... Is that why we get better by eating more plants, especially thanks to potassium intake?

Funding his research against cancer with the funds raised by research contracts with the tobacco industry, he also discovered that in smoking, the most toxic was not tobacco tar, but the CO_2 swallowed during suction!

Indeed, as well know the ecologists, CO_2 is an acidifying gas, which, in the case of smoking, attacks the pulmonary alveoli and acidifies the water of our body, as it acidifies the ocean which absorbs the CO_2 of the atmosphere. His self-funded work, like Matthias Rath and many other scientists neglected by the authorities, has led to spectacular discoveries, since his simple molecules have for 20 years slowed down or even stopped cancers, often with a remission of several years, for tens of thousands of patients.

Of course, as the Lyon study by Doctor de Lorgeril showed, cancer prevention requires a traditional Mediterranean diet and an adapted lifestyle. He also recalls that skin cancers are not caused by UV rays, since they are often located at the level of the anus, which in most people do not see the sun. Another lye from the medical authorities. There are also more and more deaths from melanoma despite illusory protection by sun creams.

Increasingly expensive but not more effective cancer treatments costs a lot to some and pays a lot for others. In France Sanofi collects 424 million per year from social security insurance, just for a drug that could be replaced by aspirin. This medicine is sold 2.26 euros in England but 37.11 euros in France, at the expense of the taxpayer. More than the power of certain lobbies, our patients die from our conformism and our inability to question a dogma that we all know to be false. Cancer is most likely a simple disease. Today cancer is thought of as an invasion by malignant and mad cells, it is treated as an enemy by surgical strikes, poisons or radiation. This dogma is false.

For example, studies show that the removal of the prostate does not change the survival of patients, and that it is dangerous. Like the 2012 study published in the famous "New England Journal of Medicine". However, mortality from prostate cancer has dropped by less than 1% in fifty years, which means not at all. These facts are camouflaged by laboratories and the government. There is no incurable disease 40 years ago, which is curable today, zero progress.

Before the war, cancer was understood by Nobel Prize winners as a disease related to diabetes. These renowned scientists understood that the cancer cell is inundated with glucose that it cannot digest and therefore it grows.

Numerous publications, coming from laboratories in different countries show that one can, in animals, stop the growth of the tumor with simple and non-toxic molecules. Yesterday also diabetes and tuberculosis were complex and therefore incurable diseases. Cancer too will become a simple and therefore curable disease.

This method begins in the USA with the general practitioner Bergson, who learns from a patient that a New York doctor was dealing with cancers successfully. He inquired and therefore began to treat his patients with lipoic acid in low doses, and with naltrexone, and published several extraordinary cases. Cases of dazzling cancers patients that live several years later, instead of the usual few months for these cases. The existence of these patients was verified by the American National Cancer Institute. But no clinical trial was started, total silence.

Doctor Schwartz gives the example of one of his patients, Antonello, who takes, in addition to the traditional treatment, and associated with a ketogenic diet, rich in fat, with little protein and no sugars, acid lipoic which he buys in Italy, because prohibited in France, and hydroxy citrate bought in France. From the start of treatment, peritoneal metastases regress, slowly but surely, and after 6 months a CT scan confirms the regression of the nodules. He is well three years later; he has returned to work.

He says that patients have introduced him to ClO2, chlorine dioxide, which adds extra punch in synergy with other supplements, which even helps to reduce cancer. On the other hand, he says that the effect decreases after 2 or 3 years ... This may be because the chlorine dioxide neutralizes vitamin C, which prevents the production of collagen and becomes detrimental in the long term.

He specifies that technically and medically, they are completely outside the rails with these methods not recognized, but which are however the only ones to work.

Other patients have made him discover methylene blue as a supplement which also has big positive effects in certain patients. For many patients, Schwartz's method saves their lives, so it is worth reading his books, in addition to the adoption of a healthy lifestyle, as described by Doctor de Lorgeril of course!□

F / Cancer according to Pr. Beljanski

According to the book of Pr. Mirko Beljanski, "Cancer: the Beljanski approach", from 2011, ISBN 978-2813202284

It is a book written by the wife of the late Pr. Mirko Beljanski, who explains his discoveries and his fight. Today she heads his Foundation. In France, after obtaining his State diploma of Doctor of Science, he was hired by the CNRS as a biologist and researcher to work at the Institut Pasteur. Mirko Beljanski encouraged his wife to pursue studies in biology, which allowed Monique to join the CNRS too.

Together, they joined the research team led by Professor Macheboeuf.

As early as 1975, Mirko Beljanski had demonstrated that any molecule with carcinogenic potential destabilizes the DNA of cancer cells and stimulates the synthesis of these DNAs. He also developed the Oncotest, a biochemical test to assess the impact of environmental molecules on the functioning of genes; and above all, proposed a new vision of carcinogenesis which was confirmed when he showed that natural extracts had the property of inhibiting the synthesis of cancer DNA and not that of healthy DNA.

He developed four extracts: three specific extracts made from Pao Pereira, Rauwolfia Vomitoria, and Ginkgo biloba, as well as very promising RNA-fragments.

Mirko Beljanski has also shown that one of the products, Pao Pereira (Geissospermum Vellosii), has a broad antiviral spectrum. He then looked into the fight against HIV, the AIDS virus.

He published 133 articles in peer-reviewed scientific journals. Over the years, an increasing number of doctors wrote to Mirko Beljanski to order and praise his products for their patients.

François Mitterrand, President of the French Republic, used Beljanski® products to control his metastases from very advanced prostate cancer. He was getting better and better and was able to finish his second term with these products when the secret was revealed in Dr. Claude Gubler's book, "The Big Secret".

Beljanski extracts are today recognized worldwide for their effectiveness:

- Pao Pereira (Geissospermum Vellosii) formerly called PB-100 (Pao Beljanski 100), now known under the names of Pao V® and Pao V FM®;
- Rauwolfia Vomitoria, formerly called BG-8 and now known as Rovol V®;
- a specific extract of Ginkgo biloba, obtained with an original method, known under the name of Ginkgo V®;
- RNA fragments known as ReaLBuild®.

Today, Mirko Beljanski's work continues in the United States where the products are produced exclusively by the company Natural Source International, Ltd. CIRIS and the Beljanski Foundation are making great efforts to continue research and carry out clinical trials in hospital settings with Beljanski extracts.

For more information there is the BELJANSKI & ASSOCIATION CIRIS FOUNDATION website https://www.beljanski.info/

This non-profit association under the law of 1901 devotes most of its budget to research and information by promoting the sharing of experiences and information to allow everyone to have the chance to benefit from Beljanski extracts, effective and non-toxic. CIRIS is committed to this strong commitment to information, help and support for patients, through the dissemination of testimonies, in particular each year during the annual CIRIS information day open to all, and through its presence at various fairs and meetings throughout France, with 2,735 members and witnesses of the Beljanski method.□

G / Cancer according to Dr. Simoncini

According to the book by Dr. Tullio Simoncini, "Cancer is a Fungus: A Revolution in Tumor Therapy", from 2007, ISBN 978-8887241082

I added this book for the simple method which would destroy tumors, by injecting sodium bicarbonate into or near the tumors. These are bathing in a very acidic environment, so the fact of suddenly alkalinizing with this powder, can suppose a shocking effect. In addition, his theory of cancer, which is of a common fungus, Candida albicans, is strangely close to the theory of the Warburg effect, having in common the fermentation of sugar.

According to the website and video in French http://www.curenaturalicancro.com/fr/

The therapy of Dr. Simoncini is explained in the video "THE FUNGAL HYPOTHESIS".

Based on years of scientific and clinical research, at the center of each cancer tumor is a common fungus, Candida albicans. The good news is that tumors can be treated with a powerful, inexpensive, readily available antifungal agent.

From a microbiological point of view, it is always Candida which invades the different anatomical parts, causing various reactions depending on the organs from which it feeds.

These behaviors are a function of the quantity and quality of the affected tissue. An organ whose connective tissue has been invaded defends itself by a cellular hyperproduction which attempts to encyst the fungal colonies which try to colonize the organism completely. This is how all the histological varieties of neoplasia can be explained and this histological variety has no influence on the determination of the cause, which is always and only Candida.

From a practical point of view, it is always the same Candida that attacks different tissues, each time adapting itself to the type of environment it finds. The species characterizations usually assigned to the different Candida (Candida albicans, C. krusei, C. parapsilosis, C. glabrata, C. tropicalis and others) underestimate the fact that they all come from a single progenitor who, when it mutates genetically to attack a host, turns itself into a particular population. (59)

RL Hopfer, for example, has found no less than four different species of Candida in a patient's post-mortem cultures of leukemia.

N. Aksoycan demonstrated that seven different Candida populations actually have the same antigenic structure.

FC Odds reports how the same Candida population was able to colonize different anatomical areas at different times.

J. Hellstein found a common clonal origin of Candida albicans in both commensal and pathogenic populations.

His book had been translated into many languages, but seems to be unavailable now. The book describes how a fungal infection always forms the basis of each neoplastic formation, and that formation tries to spread throughout the body without stopping. For the moment, the constant, uniform and relentless growth of a tumor is in no way affected by current oncological treatments. A cure rate of cancer that hovers around 7% is mentioned in books and conventional treatises despite all the tricks and distortions of the statistics. After making the necessary corrections, this returns to practically zero. The rest is propaganda for Orthodox oncology. Based on the scientific considerations in this book which demonstrate that cancer is caused by fungal masses (like Candida), sodium bicarbonate is the only useful remedy that is now available to cure the disease.□

H / Cancer and Vitamin C

According to Dr. Cathcart:

Who has treated more than 30,000 patients in his career, Dr. Ewan Cameron in association with Professor Linus Pauling (15, 16, 17) has shown the usefulness of ascorbate in the treatment of cancer; although these studies used only a maximum of 10 grams per day of vitamin C, while Cathcart and other specialists are successful with much larger doses.

Quote from Dr. Cathcart: "Large doses of Vitamin C like 1 to 10 grams per 24 hours do only limited good. But when ascorbate is used in massive amounts, like 30 to 200+ grams per 24 hours, these amounts directly supply the electrons needed to quench free radicals from almost any inflammation. "

In 1976 the results of this clinical study with 10 grams per day by IV, (15) were spectacular, since multiplying by 4 the average survival time of terminal cancer patients, some having survived 20 times longer!

Quote from this 1976 study: "The results of a clinical trial are presented in which 100 terminally ill cancer patients received ascorbate supplementation as part of their routine treatment. The average survival time is more than 4.2 times longer in subjects who received ascorbate (more than 210 days) than in controls (50 days)." [15]

Then in 1978 they did a second clinical trial [16], which gave even more positive results, but still with only 10 grams per day.

Quote from this 1978 study: "A study was done on the survival times of 100 terminally ill cancer patients who were given an ascorbate supplement, usually 10 g / day. The two patient groups were in part the same as those used in our previous study in 1976.

Survival times were measured not only from the date of "incurability", but also from the known date of first visit to the hospital for cancer which finally reached the terminal phase. Patients treated with ascorbate had an average survival time of approximately 300 days greater than that of the controls. Survival times greater than one year after the date of inability to treat were observed in 22% of the patients treated with ascorbate and in 0.4% of the controls.

The average survival time of these 22 ascorbate-treated patients is 2.4 years after reaching the seemingly terminal stage; 8 of the patients treated with ascorbate are still alive, with an average survival time after treatment of 3.5 years."

And in 1991, Dr. Cameron published his protocol (17):

"A protocol for the use of vitamin C in the treatment of cancer, developed for several years at Vale Hospital in Leven in Scotland, was presented. Clinical experience has shown that this protocol is both safe and effective. It is not necessary to follow it "to the letter", but it does provide general advice to physicians unfamiliar with this therapeutic approach. He recommends that all cancer patients treated in this way receive an initial intravenous ascorbate treatment, followed by an oral maintenance dose to be taken indefinitely thereafter. The importance of continuous administration as opposed to intermittent administration is emphasized."

Medical authorities have simply criticized the results of these studies, and no other studies have been done with large doses of vitamin C intravenously. Studies have been done by mouth, which does not have the same effect at all, due to the limitation of absorption by the intestines, preventing sufficient quantities from reaching the blood. **Why not have redone intravenous studies?**

In addition, Pauling and Cameron, as well as others using this method, have always said that vitamin C was not the only factor to change, that it was just one of the steps to take.

A large review on studies of vitamin C against cancer has just been published in Holland in 2019. (11) It explains very clearly that the oral intake of vitamin C only allows doses up to 70 times lower than intravenous, and completely limits the presence of vitamin C in the blood to 220 µM. So this is why the results of Pauling and Cameron could not be reproduced, because their method was not applied correctly, why?

Translated excerpts from the 2019 study: "This review assesses the efficacy and safety of vitamin C administration in cancer... A total of 19 studies were included...

In the 1970s, Linus Pauling, Nobel prize winner had already developed a strategy for the use of intravenous (IV) vitamin C in cancer patients [1,2]. He treated patients with advanced cancer with large doses of vitamin C and reported a positive effect on survival. However, these studies have been methodologically criticized on several aspects such as data collection and analysis. This has resulted in limited use of vitamin C in cancer patients. Other studies carried out subsequently could not reproduce these results; However, unlike the intravenous use of vitamin C by Pauling et al., in most of these studies, oral vitamin C supplementation was used [3]. Pharmacokinetic studies show however that the mode of administration makes a big difference in the maximum plasma concentration of vitamin C, and that the administration by intravenous route is much higher (up to 70 times) than after an oral intake. [4]

Maximum plasma concentrations also continue to increase as the dose of vitamin C intravenously increases, while maximum plasma concentrations are around 220 µM, even if oral doses are increased."

However, it should be noted that this review does not include any study by Dr. Rath, who has become one of the greatest specialists in vitamin C treatments.

Safety clarification according to Doctor Cathcart: "Ewan Cameron's advice against giving large amounts of ascorbate to cancer patients with extensive metastasis too quickly at the start should be taken into account. He discovered that necrosis or extensive bleeding from cancer could sometimes kill a patient with extensive metastases if vitamin C was started too quickly". [16]

Two publications by Dr. Cathcart

Title: Vitamin c, titrating to intestinal tolerance, anascorbemia and acute induced scurvy

Source http://www.mall-net.com/cathcart/titrate.html (1981)

Abstract: A method of using Vitamin C in amounts just below the doses that produce diarrhea is described (TITRATION TO INTESTINAL TOLERANCE). The amount of oral ascorbic acid tolerated by a patient without producing diarrhea increases somewhat in proportion to the stress or toxicity of his disease.

The intestinal tolerance doses of ascorbic acid improve the acute symptoms of many diseases. Lower doses often have little effect on acute symptoms but help the body manage the stress of the disease and can reduce the morbidity of the disease. However, if doses of ascorbate are not provided to meet this nutrient drawdown potential, the first local tissues involved in the disease, then the blood, then the body in general become depleted in ascorbate (ANASCORBEMIA and ACUTE INDUCED SCORBUT). The patient is thus exposed to complications from metabolic processes known to be dependent on ascorbate.

Title: Unique function of vitamin c

Source: http://www.mall-net.com/cathcart/unique.html

Abstract: Vitamin C is a reducing substance, an electron donor. When vitamin C donates its two high-energy electrons to recover a free radical, much of the resulting dehydroascorbate is re-reduced to vitamin C and therefore used repeatedly. Conventional wisdom is correct in that only small amounts of vitamin C are needed for this function due to its repeated use. The missed point is that the limiting part of non-enzymatic free radical scavenging is the rate at which very high energy electrons are supplied by NADH to further reduce vitamin C and other free radical scavengers.

In the event of illness, free radicals are formed at a faster rate than the radicals of energy electrons are made available.

Large doses of vitamin C like 1 to 10 grams per 24 hours do only limited good. However, when ascorbate is used in massive amounts, such as 30 to 200+ grams per 24 hours, these amounts directly supply the electrons needed to quench free radicals from almost any inflammation. In addition, at high concentrations, ascorbate reduces NAD(P)H and can therefore provide the high energy electrons necessary to reduce the oxygen molecule used in the bursting of phagocytes. In these functions, the ascorbate part is mainly wasted but the necessary high energy electrons are supplied in large quantities.

What makes vitamin C therapy even more useful is that it also takes over the functions of the immune system, thus working with the body's inherent ability to fight cancer cells. A study published in the Journal of Angiogenesis Research has shown that large doses of vitamin C restrict the formation of blood vessels that are used to transport blood flow and nutrients to the tumor site necessary for its growth and proliferation. [9] In addition, intravenous vitamin C improves the quality of life of cancer patients by reducing the severity of the devastating side effects that usually accompany conventional cancer treatment such as chemotherapy and radiotherapy. [10]

According to Dr. Thomas Levy

Here is what he says about vitamin C usable against cancer, which he describes as better than chemotherapy, of August 19, 2013:
"Although vitamin C is "only" an antioxidant, its unique chemical structure, closely resembling glucose, allows it to penetrate all water-soluble areas and tissues of the body, inside cells and outside cells. It really fails to concentrate in oily areas, although it may still have an antioxidant impact, as it will regenerate fat-soluble antioxidants, such as oxidized vitamin E, back to their normal donor status electrons."

Vitamin C kills cancer cells

Although vitamin C improves the health of normal cells, it increases oxidative stress inside malignant cells. In fact, all cancer cells accumulate iron and hydrogen peroxide, and vitamin C can generate highly reactive hydroxyl radicals via the Fenton reaction which can kill the cell when it is sufficiently activated.

Normal cells have only relatively little iron and practically no hydrogen peroxide, and vitamin C cannot increase oxidative stress in these cells. In fact, in normal cells, the only effect of vitamin C is a decrease in oxidative stress. In addition, when a sufficient amount of vitamin C is chronically present inside cells, they cannot accumulate iron and hydrogen peroxide, and they cannot become malignant in the first place.

If you are reluctant to treat your cancer with vitamin C only, take it with your chemotherapy. The way information is presented to the public makes it relatively rare that someone does not want chemo. Most want to "cover all the bases" and take chemo with everything they can find good, including vitamin C. Vitamin C will neutralize any chemo-toxic medication if it meets it directly in the blood, like it was snake venom or any other blood-borne toxin. However, when vitamin C is given before chemo, or several hours after chemo, it will only help. Vitamin C increases oxidative stress inside cancer cells with chemo and will therefore increase the destruction of cancer cells, while helping to repair damage caused by chemo to normal cells.

Many cases of vitamin C resolution of cancer are documented in the literature. Generally, the best effects will be obtained by infusions of 50 grams or more intravenously, or with vitamin C encapsulated in oral liposomes, several grams per day. As discussed in other articles, many cancer patients will not improve or maintain their improvements if they do not treat dental infections, especially root canal treatments, as part of their treatment protocol.

Special leukemia

Doctor Frederick R. Klenner, a few decades ago, had established a protocol against cancer, focusing on vitamin C, but not only. (I don't have the place to reproduce it in this book.) Source: http://vitamincfoundation.org
But he said then: "Vitamin C will control myelocytic leukemia with 25-30 grams orally per day. How long should you wait for someone to start a continuous infusion of ascorbic acid for two to three months, giving 100 to 300 grams per day, for various malignancies?"
And here are two more recent video testimonials of leukemia cured quickly with large doses of vitamin C, which made headlines on New Zealand television.

A rich Australian farmer, 2011

New Zealand national TV report on the case of Alan Smith, whom the doctors wanted to "unplug", and which is now in great shape thanks to megadoses of vitamin C.
His family smuggled Liposomal Vitamin C inside his room, gave him 6 grams of that per day, and before the end of one week he was out of the hospital!
Original video: http://www.3news.co.nz/Living-Proof-Vitamin-C---Miracle-Cure/ tabid / 371 / articleID / 171328 / Default.aspx
The Presenter: This is the story of a man, a dairy producer, who returned from the dead. The doctors wanted to disconnect the life support systems. But his family refused to give up. They asked the hospital to try high doses of vitamin C.
Well, as Mélanie Ribu will show you, it turned out to be a fight, because specialists did not believe that such treatment could work. But what we can say is that the farmer is no longer on the brink of death. And as his family claims, he is living proof.
Reporter: This is farmer Alan Smith, in the life support unit, just before the doctors told his family that the life support devices were going to be turned off, and that he was going to be allowed to die.

His wife: I looked at him and he seemed hopeless, he no longer gave a sign of life.

Journalist: The woman, Sonnia and the son remember what we told them. "It was all over".

His wife: He was without words and lying there, dead, when he had always been the one who could be counted on.

Journalist: Sonnia and Alan were married when they were 17 years old. They have 3 children, and the 9th grandchild was on the right track when Allan had a severe case of swine flu.

His wife: They couldn't help us in anything. The question was "what are we going to do?" And he was 56 years old.

Journalist: Alan Smith's survival has been described as one of the most remarkable, and his return to full health one of the most controversial in New Zealand's medical history. You are lucky to be alive.

Alan: I'm very lucky ...

A New Zealand policeman, in 2014

Source "Vitamin C for cancer? 'Miracle man' Anton Kuraia's highly controversial treatment"

TV channel "1 NEWS": https://youtu.be/RBMnRmbNMr0

Diagnosed with leukemia followed by chemotherapy failure, Anton Kuraia only had a few weeks to live. He started planning his funeral.

He then tried intensive injections of vitamin C. Ten months later, his cancer is still in remission. The Whangarei policeman's trip gave him a new sense of purpose and an appreciation for life.

After two months of intensive chemotherapy, there has been little improvement. He was discharged home from the hospital with weeks to live and was told that he would go into a coma and die. The 43-year-old policeman from Whangarei, father of three, was smashed.

"I remember asking my oncology doctor if there was anything I could do, anything at all. But it was clear that there were no other options and that certain death would be upon me."

Intensive chemotherapy has taken its toll and Anton has gone from 96 kg to 74 kg.

"They pushed the envelope as hard as they could. I was so sick that I lay on my hospital bed and couldn't open my eyes to see my family."

Then there was nothing more to do. After 10 weeks in hospital and two cycles of chemotherapy, Anton left on July 31 with the news that his cancer was too aggressive and that he had eight weeks to live.

Vitamin C: It was then that Anton considered other options. The role of alternative therapies in cancer treatments has always been controversial. Doctors very rarely approve them, instead, they could cautiously say that they are happy that patients are looking for other options, but when you have no more options, you try everything.

Two days after Anton returned home, Sebastian came home from school and mentioned that a friend's uncle had used a high dose of vitamin C to help fight his cancer. Uncle had seen Dr. Wojcik at the Northland Environmental Health Clinic. Anton connected to the Internet and looked for vitamin C. "I naturally looked at high dose vitamin C, therapies and supplements on the other side of the pharmaceutical barrier".

Anton's diet has undergone a major overhaul, sugar being a food to be eliminated. Fresh fruit and vegetable smoothies have become the order of the day.

The liquid form with high dose of vitamin C is 90g of clear liquid taken intravenously to bypass the intestine: "It takes 2 to 4 hours and you feel a little groggy afterwards." After 10 weeks of healthy eating and infusions - two weeks longer than the experts had given him to live - Anton felt better and agreed to have a bone marrow biopsy.

The results revealed that the cancer had decreased to less than 1%. The cancer was in complete remission. Anton describes this moment as "extraordinary and surreal".

References for this chapter:
Books by Doctor Robert Cathcart: - Curing with high doses of Ascorbic acid (vitamin C), and - Dr. med. Robert Cathcart, MD on Vitamin C - From http://www.mall-net.com/cathcart/titrate.html
Book by Linus Pauling: "Cancer and Vitamin C: A Discussion of the Nature, Causes, Prevention, and Treatment of Cancer With Special Reference to the Value of Vitamin C."
Article by Dr. Thomas Levy: Vitamin C is better than chemotherapy https://www.peakenergy.com/articles/nh20130819/Vitamin-C-better-than-chemotherapy/
His book in French published in April 2017: La Panacée originelle, la vitamin C, by Thomas E. Lévy, ISBN: 9782879090214
Nina A Mikirova, Joseph J Casciari, and Neil H Riordan. Ascorbate inhibition of angiogenesis in aortic rings ex vivo and subcutaneous Matrigel plugs in vivo. Journal of Angiogenesis Research. 2010; 2: 2. http://www.ncbi.nlm.nih.gov/pmc/articles/PMC2820478/
Anitra C. Carr, Margreet CM Vissers, and John S. Cook. The Effect of Intravenous Vitamin C on Cancer- and Chemotherapy-Related Fatigue and Quality of Life. Frontiers in Oncology. 2014; 4: 283. http://www.ncbi.nlm.nih.gov/pmc/articles/PMC4199254/
Revue 2019 PMID: 31035414 - The Effect of Vitamin C (Ascorbic Acid) in the Treatment of Patients with Cancer: A Systematic Review Gwendolyn van Gorkom

Cameron, E. and Pauling, L. Supplemental ascorbate in the supportive treatment of cancer: Prolongation of survival times in terminal human cancer. Proc. Natl. Acad. Sci. USA, 73: 3685-3689, 1976. PubMed 1068480 https://europepmc.org/articles/pmc431183
Cameron, E. and Pauling, L. The orthomolecular treatment of cancer: Reevaluation of prolongation of survival times in terminal human cancer. Proc. Natl. Acad. Sci. USA, 75: 4538-4542, 1978. PMID: 279931 https://www.ncbi.nlm.nih.gov/pubmed/279931
Cameron, E. and Pauling, L. Cancer and Vitamin C. The Linus Pauling Institute for Science and Medicine, Menlo Park, 1979. PMID: 1787808 https://www.ncbi.nlm.nih.gov/pubmed/1787808□

3. Preventing Dementias

All dementias are on the increase, like cancers, CVD or diabetes, which indicates common causes of all these epidemics of "civilization" diseases, pollution, junk food and a sedentary lifestyle, as confirmed by many specialized Doctors.

A / "Official speech" summarizes what the authorities say.

B / "Curing Alzheimer" presents the revolutionary book by Dr Nehls explaining the protocol which, since 2013 in California, has been able to reverse Alzheimer's disease.

C / "Anti-dementia nutrition" transmits information collected by Dr. Greger and his team.

D / "Schwartz's theory" summarizes his physical theory that would cause dementia.

E / "Vitamin C for the brain" recalls the importance of this vitamin for good brain health, scientific studies to support it.

F / "Pollution" recalls that poor air quality causes a large part of dementia.

G / "Meditations" points to studies that prove the benefits of relaxing and anti-stress practices.□

A / Dementias, official speech

According to the French Ministry of Health.
Source: https://solidarites-sante.gouv.fr
The World Health Organization (WHO) considers Alzheimer's disease and related diseases to be the most serious health problem of the 21st century and urges countries to see dementia as a major public health priority.

The French population continues to age, under the double effect of the increase in life expectancy and the advancing age of the baby boom generations. The share of people under the age of 20 is decreasing, while that of those aged 65 and over is increasing (18.8% of the total population in 2015). The over 75s currently represent 9.1% of the population. Life expectancy at 65 in France is the highest in Europe. In 2014, it reached 24.0 years for women and 19.7 years for men (2.8 and 3.0 years respectively, compared to 2000).

Those who are called seniors are generally in good health, even though they are frequently affected by a certain number of pathologies (sensory impairments, impaired immediate memory, degenerative diseases, particularly rheumatic, diabetes, etc.). Women often have post-menopausal osteoporosis requiring only regular monitoring or, in some cases, treatment, to prevent complications. Generally, these disorders are not accompanied by significant repercussions in their daily life. The use of doctors and drug consumption increases regularly from the age of 45, women being significantly more consumers of drugs, especially psychotropic drugs.

Part of the elderly suffers from more serious health problems, linked to the occurrence of a cardiovascular or cerebrovascular accident, cancer or a neurodegenerative disease (Parkinson's disease, Alzheimer's disease and related diseases,…). From the age of 70, functional limitations become more frequent, a consequence of a combination of physical, sensory and cognitive problems.

B / Dementias according to Dr. Nehls

From the incredible book by Dr. Michael NEHLS, only available in German or French, "Curing Alzheimer's", from 2017, ISBN 978-2330072834.

It is the first book that explains how to reverse Alzheimer's disease, and it is also very comprehensive regarding explanations of the causes of the disease. Personally it was a great opportunity to find this book, in a train station relay, because it allowed a dear person to find her memories back in just a few weeks.

Michael Nehls is a doctor and researcher in molecular genetics, former director of a biotechnology company. In his book he presents the latest clinical research - American but also European - which proves the reversibility of Alzheimer's symptoms during the early stages of the disease, when it only affects the hippocampus.

It is now known that this is where the disease begins and progresses, quickly producing its frightening symptoms (disturbances in immediate memory, loss of sense of direction, regression of cognitive faculties, etc.). These spectacular results provide proof that certain combined non-drug prescriptions (lifestyle, diet, detox, sleep, sport, etc.) not only prevent the progression of the disease, but also suppress the symptoms that have already appeared. One day, more and more patients will be able to say: I had Alzheimer's. Pleasant to read and perfectly rigorous from a scientific point of view, it offers a new look at this disease.

The method that cures Alzheimer's in California since 2013

The mainstream media do not echo it, neither the TV shows, nor the scientific magazines which nevertheless have a share of responsibility, but know that since 2013 in California, USA, clinical trials have radically improved the daily lives of 9 out of 10 patients diagnosed with Alzheimer's. [1]

Yes, 90% of people have experienced strong improvements, and even 6 out of 10 have been able to return to work! In our society still based on intensive work, it is a very strong factor of appreciation, to be able to return to work. The researchers had a systemic approach to reverse this form of brain breakdown which is considered to represent 70% of dementias. The remaining 30% is called "vascular dementia", which is therefore more directly related to a problem with the blood vessel system. [2]

This is the case of "Cerebral Amyloid Angiopathies (AAC)", a group of angiopathies (diseases of the blood capillaries) characterized by the presence of amyloid protein deposits on the walls of the cerebral vessels. The term "amyloid" is used to describe the buildup of insoluble proteins with a pleated beta configuration and a fibrillar structure. [3] They are frequent in the elderly and considered to be one of the main causes of hemorrhagic and ischemic strokes.

The medical administrations is extraordinary at naming and classifying "diseases", as we can see on one of their websites, but completely deaf, blind and mute concerning the clinical studies which have found and proven the origins and cures of these pathologies. For what reasons, I will let you answer that ... in the case that interests us, the researchers speak of dietary and behavioral "deficiencies" which prevent the renewal of neurons and normal brain cleaning. We are therefore far from a "disease", but rather from behaviors that we have that are not adapted to our cerebral physiology.

Here is one of these fine lists: from the CERVCO website (3)

Lariboisière Hospital specializes in the management of the following rare vascular pathologies of the retina, brain or spinal cord: CADASIL, familial vascular leukoencephalopathies, amyloid angiopathies cerebral, retinal arteriolar tortuosities, hereditary cerebro-retinal vasculopathies with or without mutation of the COL4A1 or TREX1 genes, hereditary retinal and cerebral cavernomas, retinal hemangioblastomas of Von Hippel Lindau disease, Moya-Moya disease, arteriovenous malformations, cerebral venous malformations familial cerebral, cerebral venous thromboses, retinal arteriovenous communications, dissections of the hereditary cervical and cerebral arteries, IRVAN, familial hemiplegic migraine, Coats disease, peripheral telangiectatic masses, macular telangiectasia and exudative vitreoretinopathy family. '

So in my opinion, and from experience, if you suffer from any ailment, get a good diagnosis from these state agencies paid by the citizens, then search a lot to find doctors or clinics aware of the solutions that exist, because you are likely to find some. Many books also present proven healings, and some are written by great doctors, from all over the world, and present thousands of testimonials, even tens of thousands of successes for certain methods discovered by medical professionals. Again, why our medical officials turn a blind eye to this evidence, I'll let you think about it.

The national medical administrative system can only direct you to surgical operations or corrosive products that will partially reduce your symptoms, without restoring the whole system of your body, this special physiology that needs essential elements in our diet and behavioral habits, which a cocktail of molecules can never replace.

There also seems to be a problem with the diagnosis itself, since they separate dementias into different groups, while they seem to have common basic mechanisms! We are told, for example, that Alzheimer's is completely different from an CAA, and yet there are excessive amyloid plaques in 70% of Alzheimer's cases! So a problem is common to them in most cases! It seems that the degradation of the functioning of these amyloid proteins, supposed to have a protective role, is at the heart of these dementias.

So, in 2013, Professor Bredesen, Dale E., (Medical Doctor and Director of Neurological Research at the University of Los Angeles) and his team…. have shown that a holistic approach to patients' lives, and the readjustment of certain eating and behavioral factors, can restore the proper functioning of the systems that regulate the brain, in particular, and allow it to regain and maintain its proper functioning until very late in human life. [5] [6]

They understood and proved that it was deficiencies and bad behaviors, essentially eating, that led to dementias like Alzheimer's and CAA.

So, once again, it all comes down to food, to the 'building blocks' that we provide to our bodies to repair themselves on a daily basis. And yes, it is not enough to count macronutrients like carbohydrates, proteins and lipids, because our body needs thousands of different and complementary small elements to properly function for all its many types of cells.

This scientific study is published free of charge in its entirety on the Internet by the newspaper "Aging", and we can therefore discover the entire protocol of the changes requested from patients, and also read the spectacular results obtained.

We note that most of the elements relate to food, and that the majority can be set up easily by an individual who would like to be cured, and a part which makes it possible to optimize the results is taken in charge by a doctor who will serve to make regular blood diagnoses and to take some medicines to maintain certain factors at an optimal level. [5]

Of course, it is in English and uses technical vocabulary, so we needed a book which explains things to us more clearly, and in French... and this was done by a great German researcher, Doctor Michael Nehls, and the book is only available in German and French. And it is in all bookstores. This very accessible book explains the why and the how of the success of this first American study, but also references and compares other clinical studies which have had more or less interesting results. There are therefore all the explanations for implementing the majority of the protocol that cures Alzheimer's, as well as very useful testimonials and additional information.

The cycle that leads to these brain degradations has been discovered, and it is from its practical understanding that the systemic protocol has been implemented, and its adaptation to respond to different important factors, allows to obtain very spectacular results. in very short times. To give you an idea of the mechanism, these are new neurons created daily in the hippocampus, which have the role of expanding memory, which die because they have become resistant to insulin, and therefore can no longer accept sugar within them as a source of energy.

The major interventions are therefore to suppress insulin spikes and provide ketone bodies to neurons as a source of energy. The results are almost immediate, because from the first days the patients show impressive improvements in their cognitive abilities. Chronic stress also plays a major role, because of the cascade of molecular reactions it causes, its management is also an essential element of the protocol. Then there is a whole series of food supplements to take, especially during the intense treatment phase, which are micronutrients necessary for the proper functioning of the nervous and cardiovascular systems.

Here are the supplements listed in the table (in order of appearance):

Vitamin B12, Curcumin and Ashwagandha, DHA and EPA, Magnesium L-threonate, Bacopa monniera, Vitamin D3 and K2, Citicoline (CDP-Choline), Acetyl-L -Carnitine (ALCAR), Red berries (for their tocopherols and tocotrienols), Selenium, Vitamin C (ascorbate), Alpha Lipoic Acid, Thiamine (vit B1), Pantothenic acid (vit B5), Resveratrol, Coconut oil.

Coconut oil is at the bottom of this list, but you will discover in the book that it is a prime factor in supplying energy directly to insulin-resistant baby neurons, because when it is taken far from meals, the liver uses it very easily to make ketone bodies, which can penetrate the cells without hindrance to provide them with clean and powerful energy ...

This book by Doctor Nehls being an analysis of several different clinical studies, we learn that other elements not used in the first Californian study are useful and effective, like the EGCG present in certain green teas from China, which helps to regulate the amyloid function and to disaggregate the toxic plaques already accumulated.

Let us fight so that our political and medical leaders become aware of these revolutionary results, and have the courage to communicate them to the people they represent and by whom they are mandated. For the health of the people we love!

References:

[1] PREDIMED study, original published NEJM - Primary Prevention of Cardiovascular Disease with a Mediterranean Diet
[2] Book Preventing vascular accidents through food
[3] Familial Cerebral Amyloid Angiopathies https://www.cervco.fr/ fr / maladie / en-savoir-0
[4] Reference Center for rare diseases of the Brain and Eye Vessels https://www.cervco.fr/fr
[5] Dale E. Bredesen, Reversal of cognitive decline: A novel therapeutic program http://www.aging-us.com/article/100690/text
[6] Long curriculum by Dale Bredesen on the site of the Alzheimer research center http://www.eastonad.ucla.edu / about-us / faculty-and-staff / item / bredesen-dale-e-md□

C / Dementias according to Dr. Greger

Here is some information presented in Dr. Greger's book "Eating better can save your life"; (old title: How not to die?).

Once again, these Alzheimer, Parkinson, Cerebral Amyloid Angiopathy (CAA), whose number of victims explodes worldwide, are strongly linked to our change in diet, which weakens our circulatory system, which results in less blood supply to the brain, and the premature death of our neurons, and an impediment of neurogenesis.

But it also causes less evacuation of the waste that accumulates there and prevents brain cells from functioning properly. We can also recall the concept of insulin resistance of neurons, by excess of sugary food, as described in the book by Dr. Nehls.

Concerning Alzheimer

According to the American Alzheimer Foundation, Alzheimer is 1,000 hours of unpaid work per year per patient, for family and friends who take care of her/him, or almost 3 hours per day. [59] Billions are spent each year on finding a solution, and 73,000 scientific articles have been published in the past 20 years, or 100 issues a day. Changes in lifestyle and diet can prevent their arrival. What is good for the heart is good for the brain, because clogging of the arteries plays an essential role in this disease too. [61,62,63,64]

According to the study of the journal Neurobiology of Aging, for the prevention of Alzheimer, as for the prevention of cardiovascular diseases and diabetes, vegetables, legumes and whole grains should replace meat and dairy products as the basis of the diet. [65 = PMID: 24913896]

Moreover, as early as 1901 in Germany, with the first case studied by Dr. Alzheimer, during the autopsy of the patient, he noted that the cerebral vessels were atherosclerotic, that is to say hard and blocked. [67 = PMID: 8713166]

Atherosclerosis affects the whole body, since we have blood vessels in all of our organs, near each of our cells to nourish them. [68]

From the 1970s the concept of cardiogenic dementia was proposed, since the brain is extremely sensitive to the lack of oxygen. Many facts today show a link between atherosclerosis and Alzheimer's. [69,70] Autopsies show that Alzheimer's patients accumulate more atherosclerotic plaques in the brain, and memory areas are severely obstructed. [71,72,73,75]

Under the electron microscope one can observe cholesterol crystals around the aggregates of amyloid fibers. PET scanners have shown a direct correlation between LDL cholesterol in the blood and the presence of amyloid plaques. [85.86]

Proof that Alzheimer's is more linked to food than to genetic inheritance, in rural India there are 3% of patients, the lowest rate in the world, among lacto-vegetarians, against 19 % in the USA, 6 times more. [90]

Alzheimer's is more common in Japanese living in the USA than in those living in Japan, the same for people in Africa or China. [91,92,94]

In populations that change their diet, from whole grains and vegetables, to dairy products and meats, this disease also explodes. Even in the USA, those who do not eat meat, poultry or fish, halve their risk of Alzheimer's, and by 3 after 30 years of vegetarianism. [98]

Of course, genetic predisposition still plays a role, because if both of your parents have the ApoE4 gene, which makes the cholesterol transporter protein in your brain, your risk is multiplied by 9. [99,100] But it's the Nigerians who most frequently have this ApoE4 gene, and yet they are among those who suffer the least from Alzheimer's. Indeed, they have a diet very low in cholesterol, very low in animal fats. [104]

Although Alzheimer's does not usually start until after 70 years of age, amyloid plaque deposits have been detected in 50% of people aged 50 and 10% of young people aged 20. [109]

Again, the Mediterranean diet is recommended for prevention. The benefits are notably attributed to the thousands of antioxidant substances that fruits and vegetables contain. [110,111,112,113]

Even fruit and vegetable juices already help, since out of 2,000 people, a 76% drop in the risk of Alzheimer's was noted. They suspect a polyphenol to be the active ingredient, although whole fruit is preferable to juice. Polyphenols could also neutralize heavy metals in the brain. [121,122,123,127,128] Gerontoxins are also to be taken into account in dementia, since they accelerate cognitive decline, by accumulating in the brain. [143,144,145]

Meat and its derivatives, exposed to dry cooking methods, and when animal fats and proteins are exposed to high heat, seem to be the major sources of gerontoxins, with tobacco smoke among others. [147,148]

Regarding Parkinson it is page 416

In addition to increasing the incidence of cancer, chemical pollutants seem to play a role in the occurrence of neurodegenerative diseases. [2,3]

The American Center for Disease Control and Prevention (CDC) regularly conducts tests on the population, and according to them, more than 99% of women are contaminated by more than 50 different chemical pollutants, heavy metals, toxic solvents, endocrine disruptors, chemicals from plastics, polychlorinated biphenyls (PCBs) and banned pesticides such as DDT. [5]

95% of the umbilical cords tested contain residues of DDT, even though this pesticide has been banned for decades in the USA. [6] And it seems that a woman's body detoxifies itself by removing pollutants from breast milk! [7,8,9] Men even have higher rates than women for certain pollutants. [10,11]

After decades of research to understand why smokers suffer less from Parkinson's, they discovered that it was nicotine that had a protective effect.

As smoking kills a huge number of people as the source of stroke and cancer, they continued to search, and it was found that protection also came from vegetables rich in nicotine, such as peppers, but only among non-smokers. This may explain the protective role already found for the Mediterranean diet, or the consumption of tomatoes or potatoes, rich in solanaceae. [58,59]

Elevated levels of pesticides and PCBs are found in the blood and brain tissue of Parkinson's patients. [60,61,62] Some of these pollutants are present in dairy products, especially cheeses, they accumulate in animal fats.

However, Parkinson's disease seems paradoxically more linked to milk and perhaps lactose, than to other dairy products. [72,73,74,75] The culprit would therefore be galactose, milk sugar described in chapter 13, which increases the risks of fractures, cancer and death. [76,77]

Dr. James Parkinson, the first to describe the disease centuries ago, noted chronic constipation until years before the disease. [101] Men who bowel movement less than once a day were 4 times more likely to develop the disease. [102]□

D / Dementias according to Dr. Schwartz

The prevention of dementia according to Dr. Laurent Schwartz

During his research, he understood that cancer was a simple disease linked to cell digestion and enzymatic defects. These same mechanisms may play an essential role in neurodegenerative diseases, such as Parkinson's and Alzheimer's.

Common points appear between cancer and Alzheimer's disease, even that of Parkinson's. All these diseases have their origin in the inflammation of the cells of the affected organs. In neurological diseases, inflammation of a specific nerve area of the brain will have its own disease. For example if it is the amygdala which is inflamed it will develop Parkinson's disease, if it is the spinal cord, it will be Charcot disease (Lou Gehrig's disease or amyotrophic lateral sclerosis).

The treatments to treat Parkinson's or Charcot or cancer will be the same, with the aim of reviving the mitochondrial activity. For thousands of incurable patients, this new way of understanding living things and diseases constitutes a bet and a great hope.

Source: Interview with Dr Schwartz on LaNutrion.fr : https://lanutrition.fr/

Is metabolic treatment interesting for all types of cancer?

It seems to me that the first real revolution in metabolic treatment concerns brain tumors, and in particular the most violent: glioblastoma. Life expectancy is a few months. The patients to whom I recommended metabolic treatment, in conjunction with conventional treatment - as long as they were in good condition, that is to say capable of taking metabolic treatment - are doing well, and this several years later.

The metabolic pathway is a promising path not only in cancer, but also in curing or improving patients with Alzheimer's and Parkinson's disease.

What to think of the ketogenic diet?

The ketogenic diet is a fundamental part of cancer treatment. Cancer is a disease of the fermentation of sugar. Reducing sugar intake and compensating for protein and fat seems important.

Source: Dr. Schwartz's page on Wikipedia
https://fr.wikipedia.org/wiki/Laurent_Schwartz_(oncologue)

Alzheimer's and Parkinson's disease are the result of increased pressure on the brain parenchyma [11,12] . This is confirmed in mice. An increase in pressure is responsible for the secretion of amyloid, synuclein or the phosphorylation of the tau protein [11,12].

The reduction in mitochondrial performance is the common point between cancer and Alzheimer's disease. Cancer and Alzheimer's disease have many things in common.

Most of the patients are elderly. More than half of cancer patients are over 70 at the time of diagnosis. Both Alzheimer's and cancer are diseases of the elderly.

Cancer like Alzheimer's disease develops more frequently on inflamed tissue. In the case of cancer, it is a chronic inflammation following, for example, alcoholism or smoking. Recently Lévy [11,12] demonstrated that Alzheimer's disease could be the consequence of inflammation caused by the heart shock wave.

(This sounds like Dr. Rath's explanation of where the cardiac arrest occurs, where the physical pulsating movement is most intense. So the dementias are due to the lack of repair in these more sensitive places due to lack of vitamin C to build collagen!?)

From a biological point of view, in cancer as in Alzheimer's disease, there is a decrease in mitochondrial activity. In Alzheimer's disease, this mitochondrial inhibition results in apoptosis, cell death responsible for neurological disorders. Recently Ms. Hamraz in her thesis defended at Paris-Cochin [22] demonstrated that the increase in pressure (caused by inflammation) inhibits the mitochondria and leads to a decrease in energy efficiency.

The central hypothesis of Dr. Laurent Schwartz is that a treatment aimed at stimulating the mitochondria can be effective both in cancer but also in Alzheimer's disease [5]. This is all the more likely since the publications show that the same molecules (lipoic acid, methylene blue, chlorine dioxide, etc.) are effective against both cancer and Alzheimer's.

Likewise, the ketogenic diet (that is to say rich in fat and low in sugars) seems effective in these two clinically different diseases.

References:

[11] - Levy Nogueira, M., da Veiga Moreira, J., Baronzio, GF, Dubois, B., Steyaert, JM, & Schwartz, L. (2015). Mechanical stress as the common denominator between chronic inflammation, cancer, and Alzheimer's disease. Frontiers in oncology, 5, 197.
[12] - Nogueira, ML, Hamraz, M., Abolhassani, M., Bigan, E., Lafitte, O., Steyaert, JM,... & Schwartz, L. (2018). Mechanical stress increases brain amyloid β, tau, and α-synuclein concentrations in wild-type mice. Alzheimer's & Dementia, 14 (4), 444-453.□

E / Dementias and vitamin C

Vitamin C and brain health

The brain is in particular need of vitamin C, as we have known since scientists discovered that the highest concentrations of ascorbate (vitamin C) in the body are found in the brain and neuroendocrine tissues such as the adrenal glands.

It seems that a chronic deficiency in vitamin C, even low, in the brain accelerates, or even causes, the onset of dementias by the formation of amyloid plaques, which could explain why the Mediterranean diet, rich in fresh fruits and vegetables, also helps prevent dementias as confirmed by Doctor de Lorgeril for example. It could also be the effect of micro-vessel atherosclerosis that takes on a special shape in the brain, using these amyloid plaques rather than cholesterol to plug the cracks.

Here is a sample of studies that explain the protective mechanisms of vitamin C for the brain, which has a major antioxidant role.

 # This 2009 study advances the importance of vitamin C against stroke and dementia.

Title: Vitamin C function in the brain: vital role of the ascorbate transporter (SVCT2). https://www.ncbi.nlm.nih.gov/pmc/articles/P

Abstract: Ascorbate (vitamin C) is a vital antioxidant molecule in the brain. However, it also has a number of other important functions, participating as a cofactor in several enzymatic reactions, notably the synthesis of catecholamines, the production of collagen and the regulation of HIF-1α.

Ascorbate is transported to the brain and neurons via the sodium-dependent vitamin C transporter (SVCT2), which causes the accumulation of ascorbate in cells against a concentration gradient. Dehydroascorbic acid, the oxidized form of ascorbate, is transported via glucose transporters of the GLUT family.

Once in the cells, it is quickly reduced to ascorbate. The highest concentrations of ascorbate in the body are found in the brain and neuroendocrine tissues such as the adrenals, although the brain is the most difficult organ to deplete of ascorbate. Combined with regional asymmetry in the distribution of ascorbates in different areas of the brain, these facts suggest an important role for ascorbate in the brain.

Ascorbate is proposed as a neuromodulator of glutamatergic, dopaminergic, cholinergic and GABAergic transmission and associated behaviors.

Neurodegenerative diseases typically involve high levels of oxidative stress and ascorbate has therefore been assumed to have potential therapeutic roles against ischemic stroke, Alzheimer's disease, Parkinson's disease and Huntingdon's disease.

This 2011 study points out the lack of vitamin C as being chronic in Alzheimer's cases, and that its antioxidant action is very beneficial on several brain biological processes, although it does not cause plaques to regress at the doses used.

Title: Vitamin C restores behavioral deficits and oligomerization of the amyloid β without affecting plaque formation in mice with Alzheimer's disease.vhttps://www.ncbi.nlm.nih.gov/pubmed/21558647

Abstract: Oxidative stress is linked to the pathogenesis of Alzheimer's disease (AD) characterized by a progressive deterioration of memory. Soluble amyloid-β (Aβ) oligomers cause cognitive loss and synaptic dysfunction rather than senile plaques in AD.

Decreased antioxidant status is associated with dementia in patients with AD, especially low levels of vitamin C.

Our group previously reported a relationship between antiaging and supplementation with vitamin C derivatives. We report here that vitamin C attenuated the formation of Aβ oligomers and behavioral decline in an AD mouse model treated with a solution of vitamin C for 6 months.

The reduction in Aβ oligomerization was accompanied by a marked decrease in brain oxidative damage and the ratio of soluble $A\beta_{42}$ to $A\beta_{40}$, a typical indicator of the progression of AD. In addition, vitamin C intake restored decreased synaptophysin and phosphorylation of tau to Ser396.

On the other hand, the deposition of brain plaque was not modified by the food intake of vitamin C. These results confirm that vitamin C is a functional nutrient useful for the prevention of AD.

This 2012 review explains its importance for cells of the nervous system that contain some of the highest concentrations of ascorbic acid in mammalian tissues. In addition to protection against stroke, and against damage after a stroke, vitamin C protects neurons from oxidative damage associated with neurodegenerative diseases such as Alzheimer's disease, Parkinson's disease and Huntington's.

Title: Vitamin C transport and its role in the central nervous system. https://www.ncbi.nlm.nih.gov/pubmed/22116696

Abstract: Vitamin C, or ascorbic acid, is important as an antioxidant and participates in many cellular functions. Although it circulates in plasma at micromolar concentrations, it reaches millimolar concentrations in most tissues.

These high cellular concentrations of ascorbate are believed to be generated and maintained by SVCT2 (Slc23a2), a specific transporter for ascorbate.

Vitamin C is also easily recycled from its oxidized forms inside cells. Neurons of the central nervous system (CNS) contain some of the highest concentrations of ascorbic acid in mammalian tissues. Intracellular ascorbate performs several functions in the CNS, including antioxidant protection, peptide amidation, myelin formation, synaptic potentiation and protection against glutamate toxicity. The importance of SVCT2 for CNS function is confirmed by the fact that its targeted suppression in mice causes generalized cerebral hemorrhage and death on postnatal day 1.

The content of neuronal ascorbate as maintained by this protein is also relevant for human diseases, because ascorbate supplements decrease the size of the infarction in stroke models by ischemia-reperfusion, and since ascorbate can protect neurons from oxidative damage associated with neurodegenerative diseases such as Alzheimer's disease, Parkinson's disease and Huntington's. The aim of this review is to assess the role of SVCT2 in the regulation of neuronal ascorbate homeostasis and the extent to which ascorbate affects brain function and antioxidant defenses in the CNS.

This 2015 study also demonstrates the importance of vitamin C in different biological processes of the brain, and that even a small chronic vitamin C deficiency has serious consequences on the formation of amyloid plaques!

Title: Vitamin C deficiency in the brain impairs cognition, increases the accumulation and deposition of amyloids and oxidative stress in APP / PSEN1 and normally aging mice.

Vitamin C deficiency in the brain impairs cognition, increases amyloid accumulation and deposition, and oxidative stress in APP / PSEN1 and normally aging mice. 2015

https://www.ncbi.nlm.nih.gov/pubmed/25642732

Abstract: Subclinical vitamin C deficiency is widespread in many populations, but its role in Alzheimer's disease and normal aging is under-studied . In younger mice, mutations with a low vitamin C content (SVCT2 (+/-)) and APP / PSEN1 increased the oxidative stress of the cerebral cortex (malondialdehyde, carbonyl proteins, isoprostanes F2) and decreased the total glutathione compared to wild-type witnesses. At 14 months, oxidative stress levels were similar between groups, but there were more amyloid-β plaque deposits in the hippocampus and cortex of SVCT2 (+/-) APP / PSEN1 (+) mice compared to APP / PSEN1 (+) mice with normal brain vitamin C.

These data suggest that even moderate intracellular vitamin C deficiency plays an important role in accelerating amyloid pathogenesis, particularly during the early stages of disease development, and that these effects are likely to be modulated by the pathways of oxidative stress.

This 2017 study focuses on the effects of aging, and shows the benefits of an adequate supply of vitamin C, with its role in protecting telomeres and the genome, and for example its anti-inflammatory effects.

Title: Vitamin C, aging and Alzheimer's disease.
https://www.ncbi.nlm.nih.gov/pubmed/28654021

Abstract: The accumulation of evidence in murine models of accelerated senescence indicates a rescue role for ascorbic acid in premature aging. Supplementation with ascorbic acid appeared to stop cell growth, oxidative stress, telomere attrition, chromatin disorganization and excessive secretion of inflammatory factors, and prolong life.

Interestingly, ascorbic acid (AA) has also been shown to positively modulate inflammatory aging and immuno-senescence, two characteristics of biological aging. In addition, ascorbic acid has been shown to epigenetically regulate the integrity and stability of the genome, indicating a key role of targeted nutrition in healthy aging. There is growing evidence in vivo supporting the role of ascorbic acid in improving factors related to the pathogenesis of Alzheimer's disease (AD), although the evidence in humans has given equivocal results.

The neuroprotective role of ascorbic acid is based not only on the general scavenging of free radicals, but also on the suppression of pro-inflammatory genes, the attenuation of neuroinflammation, on the chelation of iron, copper and zinc, and on the suppression of the amyloid beta peptide (Aβ) fibrillogenesis.

Epidemiological data linking diet, one of the most important modifiable life factors, and the risk of Alzheimer's disease is increasing rapidly. Food interventions, as a means of epigenetically modulating the human genome, can play a role in preventing AD.

The purpose of this review is to provide an up-to-date overview of the main biological mechanisms associated with ascorbic acid supplementation / bioavailability in the aging process and in Alzheimer's disease. In addition, we will discuss new areas of research and future directions.□

F / Dementias and pollution

Here are excerpts translated from the conclusions of a review study, presented in an article by the magazine Science et Avenir, "Air pollution at the origin of Alzheimer's":
https://www.ncbi.nlm.nih.gov/pubmed/30206085

Title: Are noise and air pollution linked to the incidence of dementia? A cohort study in London, Englandinvestigate

Objective: To see whether the incidence of dementia is linked to residential levels of air and noise pollution in London.

Participants: 130,978 adults aged 50 to 79 years registered on January 1, 2005, with no history of dementia or nursing home residence.
Conclusions: We found evidence of a positive association between residential air pollution levels in London and the diagnosis of dementia, which is not explained by known confounders.

Dementia, which includes both vascular dementia and Alzheimer's disease, is now reported to be the leading cause of death in England and Wales, accounting for 12% of all registered deaths.

In terms of years of life lost, the global burden of illness in 2013 ranked dementia as the fifth leading cause, noting its increasing importance as a cause of death.

Therefore, primary prevention of dementia is a major global public health problem for decades to come. For Alzheimer's disease, for example, while it has been estimated that small delays in its onset and progression could significantly reduce its estimated future burden, research has mainly focused on lifestyle factors, where a large systematic review estimated that about a third of Alzheimer's disease could be attributed to potentially modifiable risk factors such as smoking and physical inactivity.

Although air pollution is a well-established risk factor for cardiovascular and respiratory diseases.

A recent systematic review of the epidemiological evidence linking air pollution to outcomes related to dementia identified 18 studies, most of which reported adverse associations. Subsequently, a large population-based study in Ontario, Canada, reported that living near main roads was associated with a higher incidence of dementia, with further analysis revealing corresponding associations with nitrogen dioxide (NO2) levels and the mass of fine particles with a diameter less than or equal to 2.5 μm (PM2.5).

These results raise questions about the mechanisms of early development of neuroinflammation and neurodegeneration, and require further exploration and replication in other large population cohorts with different exposure patterns, including traffic noise. which has been linked to cognitive decline in adults.

Nanoparticles reach the brain via the olfactory bulb

Over the eight years of follow-up, 2,181 subjects were diagnosed as victims of dementia, or 1.7% of the sample. 39% developed Alzheimer's disease, and 29% developed vascular dementia, and 2% had both. □

G / Dementias and meditations

Scientific studies have clearly shown for several decades that the various forms of meditation and slow physical practices change the functioning of the brain, and of course also help in the management of stress, which is also a biological cause of inflammation in cells and certain organs. Cortisol is necessary but, like insulin, very corrosive to the walls of the arteries, and therefore excess should be avoided.

According to specialists, meditations act on the psyche but also on the physical body. They:
- Improve the regulation of emotions
- Improve memory
- Calm the center of fear, anxiety and stress, the amygdala
- Increase the focus of attention
- Reduce sensitivity to distraction
- Promote falling asleep, providing restful sleep, unlike sleeping pills
- Reduce the use of painkillers
- Allow to feel less pain
- Decrease relapse of depression by 50%, compared to conventional monitoring

But they also improve the expression of our genes and slow cell aging, both of which are often influenced by our stress!

Take part in the INSERM project in Caen, the Silver Health Study, on the website https://silversantestudy.fr/

Research project aimed at improving the well-being & mental health of seniors.

Participants in this study will be offered different interventions, such as learning a foreign language or regular meditation. The results will be evaluated by combining different approaches, sleep measures, reports drawn up by the participants themselves, behavioral measures, etc.

The MBSR and MBCT programs are among the most renowned. Official site: https://www.association-mindfulness.org/index.php

MBSR (Mindfulness-Based-Stress-Reduction or Reduction of Stress Based on Mindfulness) is the founding program created by Jon Kabat Zinn in 1979 'University of Massachusetts. MBSR has undergone several adaptations, the first and best known of which is MBCT (Mindfulness-Based Cognitive Therapy).

Rooted in the mainstream of integrative medicine, these protocols have allowed many scientific studies, since their origin. Due to their format, MBSR and MBCT give researchers a reliable tool on which they can rely.

These programs take place over 8 weeks, with the same group. They ask for a commitment from the participant who sets up a regular practice of Mindfulness meditation between sessions.

These programs allow learning and progressive integration of Mindfulness through meditation practices to be carried out daily, associated with yoga movements, scientific knowledge and contributions from psychology or communication sciences. The term "Mindfulness-Based" translates this complexity of elements. They integrate different approaches alongside Mindfulness meditation, the traditional practice of which is much broader than what is covered in the field and the time of an 8-week program in preset format. The main intention of these programs is above all preventive and educational. By setting up a regular practice, the participants develop their autonomy and their ability to take care of themselves, to find a better balance and a better quality of life.

MINDFULNESS AND SCIENCE: For thirty years, science has been interested in meditation and seeks to explain its cognitive and emotional benefits and, more generally, its positive impact on health. This field of research has made it possible to better explain the interconnection between the body, the mind, the brain, subjective experience and well-being. Scientists have tried to provide evidence for what contemplatives have described for millennia. This evolution of research owes a lot to the emergence of Mindfulness-based approaches that appeared in the medical sector in the late 1970s.

See the book "Brain & Meditation", By Matthieu Ricard & Dr. Wolf Singer. Source: His website https://www.matthieuricard.org/

He has been a Buddhist monk for forty years, Matthieu Ricard is a very experienced meditator, regularly contacted by universities around the world to lend himself to experiments on the brain . Neurobiologist, Director Emeritus of the Max Planck Institute for Brain Research, Wolf Singer is one of the world's leading brain specialists. For eight years, they shared their knowledge and wondered together about the functioning of the mind.

Does meditation modify neural circuits? How are emotions formed? What are the different altered states of consciousness? What is "me"? Does free will exist? What can we say about the nature of consciousness?...

Each time, Matthieu Ricard and Wolf Singer confront two traditions of thought. One, Buddhist philosophy, is first-person knowledge, the result of the millennial practices of Tibetan monks. The other, neuroscience, is third-person knowledge from laboratory experiments. The two approaches are radically different, but they often lead to the same conclusions. To develop a true "science of the mind", their rapprochement, outlined for a few years, is essential. This is what this book offers: an in-depth dialogue between the contemplative sciences and the modern sciences, in order to unravel the mysteries of the human spirit.□

4. Preventing Diabetes

Type 2 diabetes is on the rise, like cancers, CVD or dementias, which indicates common causes to all these epidemics of diseases "of civilization" or "overabundance", pollution, junk food and a sedentary lifestyle, as confirmed by many specialized Doctors.

We can quote the research by Dr. Taylor from the University of Newcastle which has inspired several books by other Doctors.

A / "Official speech" summarizes what the authorities say about diabetes and prevention, it corresponds with the results from scientific studies.

B / "The Mosley Method" presents Dr. Mosley's book and his method of getting rid of diabetes in 8 weeks or less. He uses the Mediterranean diet, physical exercise and stress reduction.

C / "Seignalet" presents Dr. Seignalet's book, and his opinion on diabetes.

D / "The 3 diets" presents a book and articles published by Thierry Souccar's very well-furnished publishing house, and the 3 recommended methods.

E / "Dr. Greger" presents extracts from Dr. Greger's book, with scientific and nutritional details, with a plant food orientation.

F / "Diabetes in neurons" mentions the explanations of Dr. Nehls on the insulin resistance of neurons which causes memory loss, and how to remedy it.

G / "Vitamin C" talks about the similarity between the glucose molecule and that of vitamin C, and the explanations of Drs Rath and Klenner on the role of vitamin C in diabetes.

H / "Some studies" presents some more scientific studies on significant discoveries in the field of diabetes.□

A / Diabetes, the official speech

The government knows well the means to prevent type 2 diabetes, more than 90% of diabetics, by changing their diet, doing physical exercise, with the need to lose weight. However, as always, citizens do not seem to be informed or do not realize how important it is not to get sick.

Source from the French Ministry of Health: https://solidarites-sante.gouv.fr/

Type 1 diabetes represents 5 to 10% of diabetes cases. It is due to an absence of insulin secretion by the pancreas. There is no known way to prevent type 1 diabetes. It usually appears in childhood or adolescence and its treatment is based on lifelong insulin therapy.

Type 2 diabetes, the most frequent (92% of cases in France), is favored by insulin resistance, that is to say a decrease in sensitivity of cells to insulin which leads to an increased need, to which the secretory cells of the pancreas end up being unable to respond.

Type 2 diabetes generally appears after 40 years, its frequency increases with age with a peak between 75 and 79 years (20% of men and 14% of women treated for diabetes in this age group in 2013).

It can be overlooked for several years. In 2006, the national nutrition and health study estimated that nearly 20% of type 2 diabetes in adults between 18 and 74 years of age were undiagnosed.

Type 2 diabetes: a global epidemic

According to WHO estimates, the number of people with diabetes in the Europe region increased from 33 million in 1980 to 64 million in 2014; type 2 diabetes accounts for over 90% of these cases. This increase in the number of cases is partly linked to aging and an increase in the population, but the epidemic is closely linked to the progression of obesity and all the risk factors linked to lifestyle habits.

Diabetes: a major risk factor for cardio-neurovascular disease

Diabetes - both type 1 and type 2 puts people at increased risk of cardio-neurovascular disease and death. It can damage the heart, blood vessels, eyes, kidneys and nerves.

Diabetes multiplies by 2 or 3 the risk, in adults, of heart or cerebrovascular accidents. It is the leading cause of blindness before age 65, the leading cause of non-traumatic amputations (rate 7 times higher in diabetics), one of the main causes of renal failure (renal dialysis rate 9.2 times higher in diabetics).

We reduce the risk of developing type 2 diabetes in the population:

By promoting a balanced diet, in particular by consuming fruits and vegetables, foods rich in fiber and by limiting the consumption of fatty products or added sugars such as sodas;

By promoting regular physical activity;

And reducing overweight and obesity.□

B / Diabetes according to Dr. Mosley

According to the book by Dr. Michael Mosley, "8 weeks to end diabetes without medication", from 2017, ISBN 979-1028503123. LEDUC editions.

Preface by Dr. Reginald Allouche, diabetologist, author of "The anti-diabetes method". Foreword by Professor Roy Taylor, a great English specialist, author of the famous Newcastle study.

The revolutionary method to get rid of diabetes is finally coming to France! Diabetes, an incurable disease? It is time to forget all these received ideas! Discover an unprecedented and proven approach to losing weight and reducing your blood glucose level. More than 3.5 million French people have type 2 diabetes. Overweight, poor diet and a sedentary lifestyle are the main source of this epidemic. In this topical book, Dr. Mosley explains why we dangerously accumulate abdominal fat and shows us how to eliminate it quickly.

A NEW METHOD THAT IS INTENDED FOR:
Those with a risk of chronic hyperglycemia. Those who want to get rid of their type 2 diabetes and stop diabetes medication. Those who want to lose weight and stay healthy.
ON THE PROGRAM: A detailed plan over 8 weeks
4 weeks of menus + 50 anti-recipes
"This book is based on the latest scientific studies interspersed with moving stories" ... It helps to better understand the biggest health problem of our time. Professor Roy Taylor of the University of Newcastle.

In the preface, Dr. Reginald Allouche, Diabetologist and nutritionist, tells us that 80% of modern diseases are due to our bad way of eating and consuming. In question the sedentary lifestyle, the excess of sugar, salt, tobacco and alcohol. Yes, our life expectancy is slowly increasing, but our healthy lifespan is declining. The French in particular spend their last 20 years with one or more forms of illness.

It confirms that type 2 diabetes, called fatty or sweet diabetes, affects all countries, poor and rich, since it is caused by artificial industrial food which is now sold everywhere, based on taste, overloaded with sugars, hydrogenated fats, salts and chemicals such as preservatives, colors, texturizers, sweeteners, etc.

In addition, during the 5 to 10 years preceding diabetes, the so-called pre-diabetic period, it is enough to lose 5 to 10% of your weight and do 150 minutes of physical activity per week to reverse the situation, and therefore avoid becoming diabetic.

We are talking about at least 1 billion prediabetic people in the world, who could easily avoid becoming diabetic, if they were informed and helped to change their lifestyle. It reminds us that type 2 diabetes ends up causing horrible complications, such as blindness, amputations, impotence, neuropathy or deterioration of the cardiovascular system, and a double risk of suffering from Alzheimer's, stroke or cancer! All of this is so easy to avoid!

It is a deep chronic inflammation that eventually destroys the entire body. It is from the impact of junk food on our liver and pancreas that it begins.

Foreword

Prof. Roy Taylor, in the foreword, explains his surprise when he discovered in 2006 that type 2 diabetes was not an incurable disease as he believed. What shocked him was the result of a study published in a scientific journal, where it was written that people who undergo bariatric surgery to fight obesity, see their blood sugar levels return to normal after just a few days, and can therefore stop their medication!

This was consistent with the theory he developed, that type 2 diabetes was simply due to excess fat in the liver and pancreas which interfered with insulin production.

And so the solution, as proven by this study on food restriction by surgery, is simply to eat less, to reduce caloric intake.

His 10 years of research with his team, show that it is possible to get rid of diabetes in 8 weeks and weight loss. His very low calorie diet has shown in several clinical studies that it works in just a few weeks.

It is the first time that humanity has been confronted with an excess of food, and in addition highly processed, and it is a major cause of our modern chronic diseases.

Introduction

He tells us that many of us are in chronic hyperglycemia, that the way we live, eat, brings us too much sugar in the blood, every day. Many do not have symptoms, but otherwise the signs are frequent tiredness, thirst and urination, and especially the small wounds which heal slowly. The latter being for me the most obvious, which still happens to me during my junk food periods.

This excess of sugar is the preliminary phase that brings us to type 2 diabetes if we stay there for years. And when our blood sugar gets out of control, that's when we talk about diabetes. Today it is a global epidemic, which is spreading everywhere and very quickly, all because of our change in diet, driven by the abundance of cheap processed food. It was because he had himself been diagnosed with diabetes that Dr. Mosley, an English doctor and investigative journalist, took care of finding a solution to it, and then published this book, which explains how to change the way to eat to get rid of it.

This book, in addition to the clear diet to follow over 8 weeks, just 2 months, contains testimonials of patients who have been cured. Hyperglycemia modifies proteins that inflame and help harden and clog the walls of our vascular system, but also damage nerves. The risk of stroke is doubled in diabetics, but also in pre-diabetics. But it is also the risk of dementia that is doubled.

Hyperglycemia also attacks the collagen and elastin molecules, which make up our skin, but also the walls of our blood vessels. This is why hyperglycemics seem much older than others.

And 70% of diabetics must take blood pressure medication, which itself accounts for 40% of the risk of stroke. And 65% of diabetics must also take cholesterol medication. It is also the number one cause of blindness, helplessness and amputation in wealthy countries. And most dialysis patients are diabetic, since diabetes causes renal failure in 50% of diabetics.

It's huge, eating less or Mediterranean resolves most ailments, and in a few weeks. The savings from health insurance would be enormous, and the contributions levied could almost disappear, keeping resources only for accidents.

Chapter 2 quotes several clinical studies. Chapter 3 teaches us that stress is an important aggravating factor, because of the cortisol cycle, which causes insulin resistance. (As Dr. Nehls also very well describes in his book "Curing Alzheimer", not yet available in English.) Many depressions are caused by this need to take more and more drugs over the years and the deterioration of the physical body.

In chapter 4 we find our famous Mediterranean diet, whose studies have shown the effectiveness to prevent cardiovascular diseases, type 2 diabetes, cancer and dementia. It's not about eating pizza and pasta, but fresh fruits and vegetables, legumes, oily fish, oilseeds and olive oil. He then tells us about the addictiveness that carbohydrates produce, and the fact that we are all potential victims.

The diet that reverses diabetes (RAD for Anti Diabetes Diet) is in the second part of the book, and recipes are also present in the third part. This diet is focused on 3 pillars, the same ones found elsewhere, that is to say the Mediterranean diet, physical exercise and stress reduction. Everything is well detailed, so make the effort to seize your chance to get better, much better, by following this guidance.

A book that can save millions of lives around the world!

C / Diabetes according to Dr. Seignalet

According to the book by Dr. Jean Seignalet, "Food or the third medicine", from 2012, ISBN 978-2268074009.

Out of 25 cases of type 2 diabetes, Dr. Seignalet obtained 20 complete remissions, and 5 improvements of 50%, ie positive results in 100% of the cases.

The Seignalet diet is therefore certainly to be implemented or added to a Mediterranean diet to quickly get rid of diabetes mellitus, known as type 2.

D / Diabetes according to the "Editions Souccar"

According to the article "3 diets that reverse diabetes" on the site of Éditions Thierry Souccar, which offers several very interesting books, written by serious doctors and scientists:
https://www.thierrysouccar.com/

Diabetes is no longer an incurable disease. Research shows that it is possible to cure it today through food. Discover the 3 most effective diets and the testimonials of patients who have adopted them.

1- The Newcastle protocol or low-calorie diet without carbohydrates

Professor Taylor and his team sought to reproduce the effects of stomach reduction surgery, but without operation. They formulated a very strict and brutal diet of 600-800 kcal (calories) per day for a few weeks. The main thing is to eliminate fats from the liver and pancreas, which cause insulin resistance. It may seem difficult to set up, due to the necessary change in diet and the sporting practice that goes with it, but it acts very quickly, with patients who come out of diabetes in the weeks that follow! And the effects last a long time, the food is pleasant and easy to find, since it is an improved Mediterranean diet.

See the testimony book of physicist Normand Mousseau "How I overcame diabetes without medication", Editions Thierry Souccar.

2- The ketogenic diet

Since diabetes is a disease of carbohydrate metabolism, it seems logical that reducing them drastically can help. Especially since the body knows how to function without carbohydrates thanks to a metabolic pathway specially designed for periods of fasting and famine: ketone bodies produced by the liver. The ketogenic diet consists of mimicking the effects of fasting in order to activate the metabolism of ketones and allow them to be an alternative fuel for cells. It is a very low-carbohydrate diet, high in fat and balanced in protein.

Several studies have looked at the effects of this diet on diabetes. They show that this diet allows you to lose weight, control your blood sugar and stop using drugs.

See Bill's testimony and the book CÉTO CUISINE by Editions Thierry Souccar.

3- The vegan diet

The Canadian Diabetic Association now recommends the vegan diet for diabetics. A vegan type diet has been successfully tested in diabetics. It consisted in eliminating all foods of animal origin (meat, cold meats, milk, yogurt, eggs, fish and seafood ...), limiting the added vegetable fats (oils, olives, avocados, nuts and seeds ...), favoring foods rich in fiber (vegetables, fruits, legumes, whole grains), choose foods with a low or moderate glycemic index as much as possible and take a vitamin B12 supplement.

References

[1] Steven S, Taylor R.: Restoring normoglycaemia by use of a very low calorie diet in long- and short-duration Type 2 diabetes. Diabet Med. 2015 Sep; 32 (9): 1149-55. doi: 10.1111 / dme.12722.

[2] Goday A, Bellido D, Sajoux I, Crujeiras AB, Burguera B, García-Luna PP, Oleaga A, Moreno B, Casanueva FF. Short-term safety, tolerability and efficacy of a very low-calorie-ketogenic diet interventional weight loss program versus hypocaloric diet in patients with type 2 diabetes mellitus. Nutr Diabetes. 2016 Sep 19; 6 (9): e230. doi: 10.1038 / nutd.2016.36.
[3] Neal D. Barnard, et al. A Low-Fat Vegan Diet Improves Glycemic Control and Cardiovascular Risk Factors in a Randomized Clinical Trial in Individuals With Type 2 Diabetes. Diabetes Care 29: 1777–1783, 2006.
[4] Rinaldi S, Campbell EE, Fournier J, O'Connor C, Madill J. A comprehensive review of the literature supporting recommendations from the Canadian Diabetes Association for the use of a plant- based diet for management of type 2 diabetes. Can J Diabetes. Published online July 28, 2016.

The testimony book of physicist Normand Mousseau, PhD, "How I overcame diabetes without medication". From 2016, Editions Thierry Souccar, ISBN 978-2-36549-206-5.

Type 2 diabetes is not an incurable disease. Discover the protocol of the University of Newcastle and say goodbye in a few weeks to your diabetes. Type 2 diabetes, an incurable disease. Really? This is not what science says or what the experience lived by Normand Mousseau shows.

When this physicist receives his diagnosis, he first defers to his doctor who advises him to eat better, lose a little weight, play sports, and prescribes drugs to lower his blood sugar. Faced with very meager results, worried about the high risk of complications (kidney and cardiovascular diseases, eye disorders, nervous damage, etc.), Normand Mousseau sets out to find a credible, science-based alternative. He discovers the protocol of Professor Taylor of the University of Newcastle (United Kingdom): a diet of a few weeks very low in calories which has healed many diabetes patients. It is this protocol that he chooses to follow. Today, he is no longer diabetic.

In this fascinating autobiographical tale, Normand Mousseau delivers an excellent popularization of the causes of the disease and the means to cure it. It is the first time that a general public book presents the protocol of the University of Newcastle and the steps to follow to apply it successfully, including recipes.

E / Diabetes according to Dr. Greger

In his book "Eating better can save your life", (old title: How not to die?), Dr. Greger devotes a 30-page chapter to diabetes.

How not to die from type 2 diabetes (page 198)
He tells the example of Milan who is better after becoming vegan. There are 2 main types of diabetes. Either your pancreas produces little or too little insulin, and it's type 1, or your body has become resistant to the effects of insulin, it's type 2.

If too much sugar builds up in the blood, the kidneys can be overwhelmed, and it ends up in the urine. Type 2 diabetes spreads very quickly in this modern world, due to a diet too rich in fats and calories, which causes rampant obesity.

In the USA, more than 20 million people are diabetic, a tripling since 1990, and more than 10 million estimated diabetics not yet diagnosed. It is 50,000 cases of renal failure per year, 75,000 amputations of the lower limbs, 650,000 cases of loss of vision and 75,000 deaths per year. [5]

Excess sugar and large amounts of insulin damage blood vessels, which can lead to blindness, kidney failure, heart attack and stroke, as well as neuropathy.

Type 1 represents only 5% of cases, and its cause is not yet defined. [6.7] Type 2, the overwhelming majority of diabetes, that's the good news, can almost always be avoided and treated with a change in lifestyle and especially diet, even if you have had it for several decades.

It all started with a study of students in 1927, when one group received a diet rich in fats (olive oil, butter, egg yolks and cream), and the others received mainly carbohydrates (sweets, pastries, white bread, potatoes, syrup, banana, rice and porridge). Within a few days the fat group saw their blood sugar levels double, much higher than the carbohydrate group. [11]

It is 70 years later that the mystery was solved. These are fats that lodge inside muscle cells and thus prevent sugar from entering them. Insulin is there to get the sugar in, but the entry message is blocked by the toxic residues and free radicals that these accumulated fats produce. MRI visualizes the fat being absorbed by the muscles, and 2.5 hours later the cells block the absorption of glucose. [12,13,14,15,16,17]

Research confirms this process, and when we reduce the amount of fat in our diet, the functioning of insulin improves. [18] Be careful, the lesions of diabetes begin even before it is diagnosed. Pre-diabetics may already have such lesions. [19,20]

90% of people who develop type 2 diabetes are overweight. [33] The more plant-based foods there are, the less diabetes there is. [36] Those who stop all meats and just keep the fish, remove 61% of the risk of diabetes, and by also removing eggs and dairy products, the risks drop by 78%.

This seems to be above all a difference in vegetable and animal fats, since even at equal weight, vegetarians have 2 times less diabetes, their cells store less fat. [37,44,45] It is even more dramatic, because for example, a saturated fatty acid from meat, eggs and dairy products, palmitate, causes resistance to insulin, while fatty acid nuts, olives and avocados, oleate, seems to protect the body. [38]

It is not only a question of eating less, but of eating better. For example, this study which added 800 g of legumes (beans, peas and lentils) per week to the diet of a group, while the second group reduced its daily amount by 500 calories, gave equivalent results of weight loss in the 2 groups.

Another study showed that a diet of vegetable origin gave better results than the diet recommended by the American association of diabetes, and it was without restriction of the quantities of vegetables and starchy foods eaten. [58]

Less cardiovascular disease also with the vegan diet. [59] Asia has a very low rate of diabetes, until a few years ago, with the introduction of western food, now it has even become an epidemic for them. In Taiwan, studying 4,000 people, they even found that occasional meat eaters, 1 serving per week for women and 2 or 3 servings for men, are twice as likely to develop diabetes. Vegetarian women had a 75% lower risk, and among the few vegetarians diabetes was nonexistent. [65,66]

The issue of nutrient deficiencies may come to mind when talking about removing meat, so a study was conducted in the US of 13,000 people. The results show, for the same number of calories eaten, that vegetarians have a higher intake for most nutrients. Vegetarians have more fiber, vitamin A, C, E, group B, B1, B2, B9, as well as more calcium, magnesium and potassium. No wonder since these very important nutrients are mostly found in fresh fruits and vegetables. In addition, vegetarians ingest less salt, saturated fatty acids and cholesterol. [74]

In several studies, diabetics who become vegetarians and gain weight still reduce their diabetes, and their need for insulin by 60%, some having no more need for it, and this after only 16 days on this diet!

Some were diabetic for 20 years and took 20 units of insulin per day and were able to stop everything after 2 weeks on the vegan diet. It is therefore never too late and it does not require you to become lean, just to stop animal fats. [99,100]□

F / Diabetes according to Dr. Nehls

According to the book by Doctor Michael NEHLS, "Curing Alzheimer", the first book which explains in detail how to reverse Alzheimer's disease, and presents the concept of insulin resistance of brain neurons, a kind of localized diabetes. Here is some information he gives on diabetes, which plays a major role in dementia.

Dr. Nehls is a former scientific director of a biotechnology company that sought to understand the mechanisms of diseases of civilization, such as CVD and diabetes, to develop drugs. It was when he started suffering from these same illnesses that he got into sport and changed his diet, and then decided to give a new direction to his career, when he saw the positive results that he was getting. So he wondered why to keep looking for drugs, when it seemed that these health problems came from a bad lifestyle.

It was after resigning from this pharmaceutical company that he decided to devote his research to Alzheimer's disease. While it was already recognized that type 2 diabetes, obesity, cardiovascular disease and many cancers were caused by poor lifestyle choices, this was not yet the case for dementias. All these diseases have progressed dramatically in recent decades, and therefore assume a common origin, such as the degradation of our environment, our food and our pace of life. Sleep is also important for staying healthy, and studies have shown a reduced risk of heart attack for people who take a nap in the middle of the day. And according to Professor Eve Van Cauter, of the University of Chicago, chronic lack of sleep causes all biological organs to age prematurely. It is also an aggravating factor for the problems of diabetes, blood pressure and memory loss.

In the chapter "Feeding the brain", he explains that excess sugar builds up on the surface of brain cells, causing local inflammation due to the immune system's reaction. These excess sugars also end up deactivating the insulin receptors of fat cells, which prevents sugar from entering and supplying them with energy, and leads to type 2 diabetes, but also to nerve cells resistance, like the hippocampus neurons needed to store new memories.

A deficiency in omega-3 fatty acids worsens this situation, since its anti-inflammatory role does not take place. This is how sugar, especially refined sugars, prevents our memory from functioning, and reduces our cognitive and learning capacities, even in children.

But so-called "trans" fatty acids also have the ability to block our insulin receptors and can be a major factor in the development of a type 2 diabetic condition. These unnatural fatty acids are present everywhere in processed foods. This is how excess sugar and "trans" fatty acids contribute to the onset of Alzheimer's disease and other dementias, by preventing neurons from feeding, which can go as far as their death.

Neurogenesis is blocked, new neurons produced every minute in different parts of the brain are prevented from developing, no longer having access to sugar as an energy source.

Type 2 diabetes or excess alcohol can cause zinc deficiency, a trace element that is very important for brain health.

The many hormones in adipose tissue, with adequate nutrition, such as leptin and adiponectin, stimulate the generation of neurons in the hippocampus, and therefore participate in good cognitive health. But as soon as there are too many fats, too much leptin is produced, and the brain's reaction is to develop cell resistance to this leptin, which blocks neurogenesis. Adiponectin on the other hand decreases in production when the fat cells fill up, and therefore too much fat still blocks the neurogenesis.

These complex and very sensitive regulatory mechanisms work very well with a natural and adapted lifestyle, but become dangerous when they are out of balance, as with our modern processed food. This excess weight, this obesity, multiplies by 2.5 the risk of developing Alzheimer's disease. But anorexia, too little fat, is also harmful, since it also prevents the stimulation of neurogenesis. Everything is in the middle ground.

In addition to reducing the consumption of sugars, and eating better, Dr. Nehls explains in his book, the method which consists in not eating for at least 12 hours each night, therefore making an intermittent fast daily, and to take 1 or 2 spoons of virgin coconut oil, in the middle of the night, or away from meals, because it contains medium-length fatty acids, which the liver can easily transform into ketones, that resistant brain cells insulin can use as an energy source. And so the new neurons can grow and start working again.

A method that works very well and is essential in the healing method of Alzheimer's disease.

G / Diabetes and vitamin C

Dr. Rath, a great specialist on vitamin C, having worked with Professor Linus Pauling talks about diabetes in his free downloadable book, which also contains testimonials:

In chapter 7, p 147 http: // www.dr-rath-foundation.org/wp-content/uploads/2018/07/pourquoi-les-animaux-07-fr-diabete.pdf

We can end these deaths in masse: According to WHO, more than 900,000 people die from diabetes each year. The sum of the "years of life lost" due to death or disability - the size of the expenses borne by the community - is equivalent to more than 15 million years of life. Source: WHO, World Health Report, 2002.

The body's confusion between vitamin C and sugar molecules is the cause of diabetic-like cardiovascular disease. The key to understanding the vascular complications of diabetes is to look at the level of molecules. The glucose and vitamin C molecules have a very similar structure, which in diabetics causes confusion in their metabolism. The consequences of this confusion are catastrophic. What happens at the cell level is summarized on the following pages.

Vitamin C lowers blood sugar and lowers the need for insulin. Clinical studies show that, in diabetics, vitamin C not only prevents the appearance of cardiovascular complications, but also helps to correct the imbalance in glucose metabolism.

Professor Pfleger and his team from the University of Vienna have published the results of a remarkable clinical study. It shows that diabetic patients who consume 300 to 500 mg of vitamin C per day can significantly improve their glycemic control. The blood sugar level can be reduced by an average of 30%, the daily insulin requirements by 27% and the sugar level in the urine can be reduced almost to zero.

More Vitamin C, Less Insulin

Diabetic patients can reduce their daily insulin needs significantly by increasing their intake of Vitamin C. This is the result of a study conducted at the famous Stanford University in California.

Dr. Dice, the main author of this work, was the diabetic subject of this case study. At the start of the study, he injected 32 units of insulin per day. During the three weeks of the study, he gradually increased the daily consumption of vitamin C to reach 11 grams per day on the 23rd day. Vitamin C was consumed in small doses throughout the day to promote its absorption by the body. By the 23rd day, his insulin requirements had reduced from 32 to 5 units per day. For each additional gram of vitamin C, Doctor Dice was able to save 2.5 units of insulin.

Crimes against humanity

It is surprising to note that the studies described above were carried out decades ago, but that, to date, almost no one knows of their existence. The investigation of Dr. Pfleger from the Vienna University Clinic was already published in 1937 in the medical journal "Wiener Archiv für innere Medezin", just before the Second World War. The Stanford University study was published in 1973, over a quarter of a century ago.

Since 1937, it has therefore been established that vitamin therapy is the basic treatment for diabetes. All of humanity would have had good reason to rejoice in this medical discovery. And yet this was not the case. The medical advances in vitamin therapy and diabetes have not been the subject of further research and have therefore not been put into practice clinically. For this reason, in the past 50 years, millions of diabetics have died from a heart attack or stroke that could have been prevented. Millions of diabetics have been blind, disabled by amputations that could have been spared them, or had to undergo dialysis due to kidney failure.

Who is responsible for this drama? Mainly the pharmaceutical industry which, to guarantee a multi-billion dollar pharmaceutical market through the treatment of diabetes, boycotted any treatment based on vitamins or other non-patentable natural products. Thus, neither doctors nor patients have been able to take advantage of vitamins to prevent and treat diabetes.

Diabetes According to Dr. Klenner

Dr. Klenner had also used vitamin C for his diabetic patients in the last century, and this is what he said. Source http://vitamincfoundation.org/www.orthomed.com/klenner.htm

These reviews have overlooked the person with diabetes mellitus. The amount of oxalic acid found in the diabetic patient is close to that found in the urine of a normal person taking 10 grams of vitamin C per day. In the diabetic, we find a paradox. Give this individual 10 grams of ascorbic acid per day, orally, and the urinary excretion of oxalate remains relatively unchanged. Diabetics are known for their diuresis. The individual who takes 10 grams or more of vitamin C each day will find that this organic compound is an excellent diuretic. No urinary stasis; no urine concentration.

Dr. Klenner says of himself: "I have taken 10 to 20 grams of ascorbic acid per day since my last visit to this college - 18 years ago. I don't have diabetes mellitus and, if I can walk away for a moment, I haven't had kidney stones either."

Response of diabetes mellitus to 10 grams of oral ascorbic acid

For the past 17 years, we have studied the effect of 10 grams orally in patients with diabetes mellitus. We found that every diabetic not taking a vitamin C supplement could be considered to be suffering from subclinical scurvy. Because of this, they find it difficult to heal wounds. The diabetic patient will use vitamin C supplementation for better use of their insulin. It will assist the liver in carbohydrate metabolism and restore its body to heal wounds like normal individuals. We have found that 60% of all diabetics can be controlled with diet and 10 grams of ascorbic acid per day. The other 40% will need significantly less needle insulin and oral medication.

H / Diabetes, some more studies

Here are some published scientific studies on diabetes

Curing type 2 diabetes is possible easily, since the scientists of the team of the famous Professor Taylor, finally found the cause, in 2016 at NewCastle University.

It occurs when the pancreas contains too much fat (triacyglycerol type) and can therefore no longer function normally to produce insulin.

It's very simple but it had to be found. It takes just 0.6 grams of excess fat in the pancreas to trigger type 2 diabetes.

This explains why scientists still find a link between diabetes, diet and being overweight. This is why there were also differences in reactions to diets between individuals, since each person synthesizes fat, preserves it and burns it under different conditions.

It was the University of Newcastle, England, who announced this major discovery on December 1, 2015.

So just lose body weight until the pancreas loses about 0.6 grams of fat (less 1 gram), so that type 2 diabetes disappears. A serious diet with physical exercise should therefore be enough to save the millions of people who suffer from it.

Here is the scientific article published on the website of the Institute of Diabetes: http://care.diabetesjournals.org

Title: Weight loss decreases excess pancreatic triacylglycerol specifically in type 2 diabetes. 2016

https://www.ncbi.nlm.nih.gov/pubmed/26628414

OBJECTIVE: This study determined whether the decrease in pancreatic triacylglycerol during weight loss in type 2 diabetes mellitus (T2DM) simply reflects body fat or specific to diabetes and is associated with the simultaneous recovery of the secretory function of insulin.

CONCLUSIONS: The drop in intrapancreatic triacylglycerol in T2DM, which occurs during weight loss, is associated with the condition itself rather than a decrease in total body fat.

In 2014 an Italian review several studies confirm the benefits of the Mediterranean diet to prevent or treat diabetes type 2.

Title: Mediterranean diet and type 2 diabetes.

https://www.ncbi.nlm.nih.gov/pubmed/24357346

Abstract: The consumption of certain food components is favorably associated with the prevention of type 2 diabetes, but discordant results for certain foods or certain nutrients continue to appear . The study of complete dietary patterns represents the most adequate approach to assess the role of diet on the risk of diabetes.

The term "Mediterranean diet" essentially refers to a diet mainly based on plants, greater consumption of which has been associated with higher survival and lower all-cause mortality.

At least five large prospective studies report a significantly lower risk of type 2 diabetes in healthy people or in at-risk patients with the highest adherence to a Mediterranean diet. Five randomized controlled trials evaluated the effects of a Mediterranean diet, compared to other commonly used diets, on glycemic control in subjects with type 2 diabetes. The improvement in HbA1c levels was greater with a Mediterranean diet and ranged from 0.1% to 0.6% for HbA1c. No trial has reported worsening glycemic control with a Mediterranean diet. Although no controlled trial has specifically evaluated the role of a Mediterranean diet in reducing cardiovascular events in type 2 diabetes, there is evidence that post-infarction or high-risk patients, including diabetic patients, may have cardiovascular benefits from a Mediterranean diet.

Evidence accumulated so far suggests that adopting a Mediterranean diet can help prevent type 2 diabetes; in addition, a low-carb Mediterranean style diet seems good for reducing HbA1c in people with diabetes.

In 2010 an Italian review of 17 studies and 5 clinical trials, confirms the benefits of the Mediterranean diet to prevent or cure type 2 diabetes.

Title: Prevention and control of type 2 diabetes by the Mediterranean diet: a systematic review.

https://www.ncbi.nlm.nih.gov/pubmed/20546959

Abstract: We carried out a systematic review of the available studies which evaluated the effect of a Mediterranean diet in type 2 diabetes. searches in publications up to November 30, 2009.

Seventeen studies were included. Two large prospective studies report a considerably lower risk (83% and 35%, respectively) of type 2 diabetes in healthy people or in post-infarction patients with the strongest adherence to a Mediterranean diet.

Five randomized controlled trials evaluated the effects of a Mediterranean diet, compared to other commonly used diets, on glycemic control indices in subjects with type 2 diabetes.

Improving fasting blood sugar and HbA1c was higher with a Mediterranean diet and ranged from 7 to 40 mg / dl for fasting blood sugar, and from 0.1 to 0.6% for HbA1c. No trial has reported worsening glycemic control with a Mediterranean diet.

Two controlled trials in a secondary prevention setting demonstrated that post-infarction patients, including diabetic patients, had cardiovascular benefits from a Mediterranean diet. The evidence accumulated so far suggests that adopting a Mediterranean diet can help prevent type 2 diabetes, and also improve glycemic control and cardiovascular risk in people with established diabetes.□

5. Preventing Depression and Suicide

It is the fifth cause of mortality in this world. On no official site have I found a mention of food or environmental pollution as factors of depression or suicide, while scientific facts prove these strong links. In particular by the fact that the bacteria in our intestines produce neurotransmitters and other molecules which influence our mood and our physical well-being. And certain strains, more often from or feeding on foods of animal origin, release aggressive products which cause brain inflammation.

A / "Official speech", presents the little information found on the official sites.

B / "Dr. Seignalet" mentions the high success rate that he had against depression.

C / "Dr. Greger", demonstrates by scientific facts the cause and effect relationship with food.

D / "Dr. Mosley" recalls that being sick is an important cause of depression.

E / "EMDR", presents a simple technique which makes it possible to reduce the incidence of past emotional trauma.

It is also scientifically established that food toxins or air pollution have effects on our psychological balance. So why is it not mentioned in these documents from health authorities? To prescribe more pills with catastrophic side effects that generate other health problems, which themselves cause the prescription of new pills in addition? It is still shocking that health officials do not know the real causes of the diseases that scientific studies have identified, right?□

A / Suicide, the official speech

Information from the official WHO site
https://www.who.int/topics/depression/en/
Depression is a common mental disorder characterized by sadness, loss of interest or pleasure, feelings of guilt or self-worth, disturbed sleep or appetite, tiredness and problems with concentration.

Depression can persist or become recurrent, thereby significantly impeding an individual's ability to function at work or school or to cope with their daily lives. At its peak, it can lead to suicide.

Information from the Department of Health Canada website
https://www.canada.ca/en.html

Causes of Depression: Major depression is a multifactorial disease. Some are genetically predisposed to depression and several external factors can increase the risk:
- The death or illness of a spouse, friend or family member;
- Difficulties at work or in a personal relationship;
- Low self-esteem;
- Financial difficulties;
- Addiction issues.

Some people experience seasonal depression at the same time each year, usually during the winter when natural light is scarce.

Hormonal changes in women can lead to depression during menopause or after childbirth.

Overcoming Depression

Depression is a treatable disease. The first step in the recovery process is to recognize that it is an illness and not a sign of personal weakness. For many people who are depressed, knowing that they are not alone, that they can get help is often enough to start the healing process.

As each person is unique, the approaches to recovery are diverse. The most frequent and effective treatment is the combination of psychological consultations and antidepressant drugs. Support from family, friends, colleagues and self-help groups can also be instrumental in recovery.

B / Suicide according to Dr. Seignalet

Here are the results of Dr. Seignalet in terms of depression, according to his book:

Endogenous nervous breakdown: on 30 cases, 25 complete remissions, 5 clear improvements, and no failure, ie positive results in 100% cases.

Migraines: out of 57 cases, 41 complete remissions, 12 clear improvements, and 4 failures, ie positive results in 93% of the cases.

Tension headache: out of 15 cases, 11 complete remissions, 3 clear improvements, and 1 failure, ie positive results in 93% of cases.

C / Suicide according to Dr. Greger

Dr. Greger devotes chapter 12 of his book "Eating better can save your life", to suicidal depression.

He recalls that food plays an important role in mood, and begins by telling the story of Margaret, who had been diagnosed as depressed at the age of 10, already suffering from suicidal thoughts and dreams on a daily basis. She was hospitalized several times during her life for depression, until she attended a conference with Dr. Greger. With the encouragement of her psychiatrist, she changed her diet, turning to whole plant products, and her condition has radically reversed, since she has not suffered from depression at all for 9 years at the date of her letter of testimony.

In the USA almost 40,000 people commit suicide each year. Major depression is one of the most common mental illnesses, more than 15 million people suffer from it in the United States alone. Mental health plays a role in physical health because happier people have healthier immune systems. Many molecules can affect the brain and the body in general, causing inflammation that disturbs well-being, such as arachidonic acid found mainly in animal products, in chicken and eggs.

Several large studies in the USA have shown a significant improvement in mood, emotional state, depression, fatigue and anxiety, switching to a diet based on plant foods.

This can reach up to minus 60% depression for fruit and vegetable eaters.

It has been shown that many elements in plants block certain neurotransmitters which unbalance the neurological state of the brain.

For example, since the 1970s it has been discovered that the lack of the amino acid tryptophan makes you irritable. It is indeed one of the components of serotonin, the hormone of happiness, which we manufacture in our brain. The positive effects on the brain and mood of the antioxidants found in fruits and vegetables could not be obtained by taking the same antioxidants in pill form.

We also know that a number of beneficial neurotransmitters are produced by bacteria from our microbiota that feed on plant fibers, which will multiply the benefits of eating plants. The folates present in green vegetables have also shown an anti-depression effect.

Another study of 100 men over 1 year, showed that those who ate the most carbohydrates, compared to those who ate less, suffered less from mood problems, depression or aggression, which was confirmed by other studies around the world.

Exercise is also recognized as effective in improving mood and reducing depression. In the USA, a study of 5,000 people, focusing only on regular physical exercise, has already noted 25% less depression among athletes. Other studies have found that exercise is equivalent to depression medication.

D / Suicide according to Dr. Mosley

Dr. Mosley explains well in chapter 3 of his book "8 weeks to end diabetes without drugs", that being sick, with always more drugs to take over the years , and because of the other side effects, causes depression in many patients, who lose all hope for a better future.

A change in diet leads to a better mood, which improves even more after the addition of physical activities, in particular by the production of hormones of well-being, then when the body needs less medication…

E / Suicide according to Dr. Roques

The books by Dr. Jacques Roques, "Discovering EMDR (Personal development and support)", of 2012, ISBN 978-2729612153, and "Healing with EMDR. Treatment, theory, testimonies ", of 2007, ISBN 978-2020881241.

Presentation of the editor

Yes, we can cure definitively, and in some cases, very quickly, a serious psychological problem. Many people have had their lives transformed thanks to this therapy invented in 1987 in the United States by Francine Shapiro.

EMDR is not a passing fad, but the expression of a major discovery: our brain is naturally equipped to heal from its psychological wounds. It can heal. EMDR is only the means by which the process of reprocessing information blocked on the day of the traumatic event can be restarted.

Jacques Roques wants to shed light on this mechanism. He gives many examples of pathologies: simple traumas, complex traumas and also mental poisonings, when the trauma, distilled in small doses like a venom, is revealed only during therapy. Based on the clinic and on what we know today about brain functioning, Jacques Roques develops new hypotheses to understand these pathologies, as well as the functioning of EMDR, to improve the care of patients and allow them to recover their health even faster.

Written in simple language, giving voice to his patients as well as to his colleagues, Jacques Roques seeks above all to disseminate useful knowledge. How can we accept that today so many people continue to suffer when they could be permanently cured?

Jacques Roques, psychoanalyst, practiced hypnosis, psychodrama and family therapy, in the office and in the hospital. Trained at EMDR in 1994, he is vice-president of EMDR-France, president of the Center for the treatment of mental trauma and the Languedoc-Roussillon Victimology Institute. He is the author of EMDR, a therapeutic revolution (2004). A book that explains very simple and effective techniques to work on psychological trauma,

EMDR therapy is a new method of psychotherapy which uses sensory stimulation on both sides of the body, either by the movement of the eyes or by auditory or skin stimuli , to induce rapid resolution of symptoms related to past events. This book provides access to a fair and complete knowledge of EMDR: its origin, its principles, its usefulness, its basic exercises, its indications and contraindications, its "good addresses" ...□

Conclusion

From the 1940s to the 1960s, doctors went to observe the populations of non-modernized countries on all continents. Their conclusion was that these populations had no cardiovascular problems, no cancers, no diabetes, no dementia, while these chronic diseases were already developing massively in more industrialized and urban countries. Then they found that these healthy people, when they migrated to a modern country, started to develop these chronic diseases. It was already proof that these ailments were not hereditary or genetic, but only due to the environment in which the person lived. Air pollution was still quite low compared to today, there were far fewer people on Earth, and fewer industries, polluting vehicles, and therefore there were two possible factors to cause these diseases, food or sedentary lifestyle, or both at the same time.

It had therefore been discovered that healthy humans eat large quantities and varieties of plant products, and animal products in limited quantities. It is generally not by ethical or taste choice, but simply because the environment in which we live determines what is available to us as a source of food. For millennia we had easy access to many vegetable products at hand, fruits and vegetables of all kinds, which we ate without overcooking them, and animal products were more difficult to access. Today it is very different, in industrialized countries we have all kinds of cheap animal products available, while fruits and vegetables are more expensive and difficult to find. In addition, we have developed all kinds of cooking habits to enrich our palette of flavors, to the detriment of the beneficial molecules present in fresh products.

The most dramatic for our body is certainly the trivialization of very industrially processed products, which are empty of beneficial micronutrients, but which in addition contain molecules indigestible by our microbial flora, which cause chronic inflammations in our intestines, which ends up unbalancing our whole organism. It is food from which our body cannot extract anything useful, but which in addition ends up becoming harmful and making us sick.

Our cells are very complicated organisms that need hundreds of different molecules to function properly. Likewise for our microbiota, which is responsible for producing many molecules that we need, but which also needs varied and specific food. Our diet must absolutely include many more elements than the 3 macronutrients and the few vitamins and minerals that we have been talking about for decades. It turns out that plants from nature are the only ones that offer sufficient complexity to meet the demands of our cells and our intestinal fauna, to nourish and protect them.

Since these discoveries no government has taken the lead in seriously studying nutrition or the need for physical exercise, they have all decided to develop allopathic medicine, to treat the symptoms of these diseases with technological science, instead of bringing society back to nutritional practices equivalent to those of less artificial populations, who are still in good health. The problems have therefore only worsened, city dwellers becoming more and more sedentary, air pollution increasing, and food becoming more and more synthetic and absorbed in ever greater quantities. Many doctors looked for alternative solutions, and when they found them, were systematically stopped as soon as they reached a certain popularity. Many were put in prison, ruined or murdered, while the patients they had cured protested or petitioned for their release, to no avail.

In 1990, the Lyon INSERM study (Lyon Heart Study) by Dr. de Lorgeril and his team, showed in a definitive scientific way to what extent diet could reduce cardiovascular diseases and cancers. Science had spoken, and spectacularly, with a result of 75% less recurrent heart attacks, just by changing food, adopting a traditional Mediterranean diet.

It was therefore to be expected that these ailments would decrease in the population, since the medical and scientific authorities now undoubtedly knew how to prevent them, at least in part. Until these indisputable results, the medical authorities still benefited from the presumption of innocence, the presumption of ignorance, or the benefit of the doubt for lack of scientific evidence. Yet the rates of chronic disease continued to rise.

We have seen that the official websites of these medical authorities explain that these diseases can be prevented by changing our lifestyle, by quitting smoking, drinking alcohol, eating too much, and by eating more fruits and vegetables, and doing physical exercise. So they know and they share information with their citizens to a certain extent.

But when we ask any random person if they know that they will be able to avoid having a cancer or a stroke, they answer that it is impossible to prevent it, that if we could avoid it, everyone would know it. And above all she/he will tell us "if it was possible to avoid cancer, my doctor would have told me about it".

And yes, this is where the flaw lies, all the information on preventing chronic diseases exists and is presented on government websites and in scientific journals, but the medical profession is completely ignorant of this data!

Whether it is at the general practitioner, at a specialist, or at the hospital level, none of these health personnel is trained in nutrition, and in the fact that it is the major factor to implement for good health. On the other hand you will be prescribed all kinds of pills and surgeries, telling you that it is the only known solution against your disease.

In the media and in scientific researchcircles it's the same, you will be told there that the solution will come from the discovery of new molecules that will cure these epidemic ailments, and that it would be enough just to give more funding to research to finally figure out how to cure the millions of people who suffer and die prematurely.

There is therefore a broken link in the information transmission chain, those who care do not know the right method to apply, which would be to change the lifestyle of their patients, and especially their diet and their amount of daily physical activity.

The overwhelming conclusion, for me, is that the people to whom humans delegate responsibility for their health, without any other legal possibility anyway, since not having the choice, are either incompetent since decades, since having neglected to integrate the results of the Lyon study into their teaching in the medical professions, or are either dishonest, because having deliberately concealed this information.

A major problem in this centralized and imposed healthcare system is the fact that huge private for-profit financial interests have the right to intervene and influence lawmakers, politicians, scientists, medical professionals, etc... What about the good of the citizens if the hungry for profit have the power to change the laws and rule the world?!

The actors of the chemical industry, with the support of our govern-ants and the bankers who finance them, for reasons they know well, it seems, have decided to artificialize us. In agriculture they have short-circuited natural processes to grow plants from poorly diversified chemical fertilizers. As a result our soils have become depleted while being over-exploited, and therefore farmers have had to use other artificial chemicals to protect plants made vulnerable by poor soil inputs and biodiversity.

The most shocking thing is that they decided to do the same with our biological bodies. They depleted our diet by focusing on 3 macronutrients and a few micronutrients. As a result our bodies have weakened, like agricultural soils, and we have therefore become much more vulnerable to diseases, like the agricultural plants. What they decided to compensate, not by better nutrition, but by giving us chemical molecules from their manufacture, antibiotics in particular, such as pesticides and herbicides for agricultural plantations. Then, this impoverishment of our organisms triggered epidemics of systemic imbalances, which they more or less control with other chemical molecules of their manufacture.

While the majority of these imbalances in our organisms did not exist, or still do not exist in populations that still eat naturally, based on rich and varied plants. These new diseases, which have been exploding for only a few decades, are moreover called "diseases of civilization"... and perhaps we should rather call them "diseases of chemical industrialization". To solve the original problem, the nutritional deficiencies in micronutrients accumulated over years, instead of resorting to this artificial chemical dependence, we just have to go back to the way of eating of our ancestors, which humans had just before this depleting chemical era.

Of course, no one bears all the fault, because many of us have chosen this way of industrial food, through our choice of lifestyle. But know that it is never too late to turn around and regain good health by starting to eat and live healthy. Furthermore, this artificialization now seems to extend to our psychology, and to our sociability, making us go through artificial electronic interfaces and virtual connection networks, to communicate and interact between ourselves.

Here again, our nature is physical, visual and auditory contact, and this artificialization will necessarily impoverish us at these levels, which will have to be more and more compensated by chemical molecules, antidepressants, alcohol, hallucinogenics and others, which are themselves also, produced by this chemical industry ... think about it! Make your choice, a return to healthy nature, or an imbalancing artificialization?

But this book is not written to target the causes of ignorance by the citizens, nor on the dishonesty of the decision-makers, but to give the keys which make it possible to find and maintain a good health, at the lesser cost, and without drugs. This system which industrialized the generalized disease will end up by dismantling itself, when the population will have found its state of natural good health.

As you have read, what we put in our body is essential for our good health, and the modernization of food, its unreasonable industrialization, as well as its large distribution requiring ever longer storage times, have pushed to produce foods empty from essential micronutrients, focusing only on flavor, visual appearance and the 3 macronutrients, carbohydrates, proteins and fats.

Today many foods available are even harmful, since they are indigestible and full of synthetic molecules unknown to our cells and our microbial fauna, which accumulate untreatable waste in our deep tissues. These manufacturers of fake food will also have to close shop or evolve, when people have changed their eating habits, after having read this seismic information, and taking over responsibility for their good health.

This book ends with a summary of the right way to "eat and move", then a few pages of reference on the actions to take to find the path to a happy life because being in good physical and mental health.

It is never too late to start living well, as numerous testimonies in these books from doctors who know how to care for you, from these people who had been condemned to a few weeks of life, and who are still with us, several years later. Your chance is there, seize it!□

The Ideal Diet

Warning: This chapter and this book do not constitute medical or dietary advice, but my personal opinion and what I would do for myself after reading all these books written by Medical Doctors and Qualified Nutritionists. Only qualified and licensed doctors and nutritionists-dietitians are entitled to advise you on diet for health, so consult them before making any decision.

According to the books of nutritionist in hospital Marie-Laure André and Dr. de Lorgeril, initiator of the Lyon Heart Study, the traditional Mediterranean diet is the most suitable because it is rich in plant products, fruits, vegetables, legumes, and cereals, and therefore fiber, antioxidant compounds, vegetable fats, and poor in animal products, meats, cold meats, dairy products and processed foods, and helps prevent, in particular, about 80% of cardiovascular disease.

The EPIC study, started in 1992 presents the same findings, and specifies that it was in the 1960s that scientists knew that food was essential; "Ecological evidence in the 1960s suggested that the traditional Mediterranean diet could have beneficial health effects".

Prior to the promotion of the Mediterranean diet, Dr. Seignalet had managed to cure many people with a similar diet, very rich in fresh or undercooked vegetable products, but which in addition had to exclude all dairy products and cereals to have final results, except rice and buckwheat. It is more than 91 diseases that respond to his diet, so it is very important to take this into consideration.

The big "China Study", by Pr. Colin Campbell, started in 1980, also concluded that the diets low in fat and rich in dietary fiber and vegetable matter, which contrasts sharply with the diets rich from western countries, were multi-protective for health. But in addition, this study shows that any intake of animal products has a negative influence on general health. (I did not have the space to summarize this study in this book because it already seems too long!)

Dr. Greger also, among others, provided in his book, number of additional arguments from epidemiological studies , clinical and laboratory, showing the harmfulness of animal products on health, even in small quantities.

Personally, I am not a vegetarian, and I think that among our ancestors, there were few vegetarians, at least by choice. But it is true that in view of these multiple scientific findings, I minimize my consumption of animal products, and much more that of processed animal products!

On the other hand, Dr. Nehls shows in his book the importance of omega-3 fatty acids for the health of our brain, and I therefore encourage myself to eat fish and seafood more often, because it is much more difficult to assimilate omega-3 from plant products. Fish has almost become the only animal product I eat.

Remember here that the amount of food absorbed is also essential. Our liver having a very limited processing capacity, as soon as it is saturated, it produces a lot of fat to send to storage. The food rations of healthy people, and therefore those of our ancestors for thousands of years, were much smaller than ours. It was also common to eat only once a day in agricultural circles, which however required great physical efforts all day. Only the rich people ate 3 times a day, and they paid dearly for it, developing all these chronic diseases almost unknown in poor households.

There have been many other studies published over the past few decades on the health benefits of diet against disease, but the selection above is far enough to validate this point.

So, I switched to the Mediterranean diet, made of unprocessed and undercooked products, and improve it further according to the results shared by these doctors. For lunch I eat a large varied salad and a smaller meal with fish in the evening. I satisfy my taste buds for happiness and the nutritional needs of my body, so we are both in great shape!

Note on vegetable juices:

For people who want to remineralize quickly, to stock up on beneficial minerals and antioxidants, I should quickly mention fresh vegetable juices. For years I have been regularly making vegetable juices, with a juice extractor, because in this way I ingest the micronutrients present in a kilo of fresh vegetables in a few minutes, which would be impossible for me to chew and get into my stomach. The molecules found in vegetables are extracted and concentrated in the juice, and are quickly absorbed into the blood, without the disadvantages that would be caused by the large amounts of fiber associated with it in the form of the whole vegetable.

Let's not forget that this is not recommended with fruits, because fruit juices are worse than sugary water, containing massive doses of fructose, which the liver massively transforms into fat to be stored. Fruits contain a lot of sugar, so they should only be eaten whole, with the fibers they contain, which allows a slow absorption of these sugars. Vegetables, especially green, containing mostly little sugar, do not produce this danger of sudden peaks of large amounts of sugar passing into the blood.

Note on the ketogenic diet:

Dr. Schwartz mentions advising the ketogenic diet to his cancer patients, and Dr. Nehls mentions its interest in the fight against diabetes and dementias. My dear Mom has also recovered her memory after only 1 week practicing the night fast of Dr. Nehls, by not eating for at least 12 hours per night, with 1 spoonful of coconut oil in the middle of the night, that the liver transforms from fatty acids into ketones which then nourish the insulin-resistant neurons in the hippocampus and other areas of the brain where neurogenesis occurs.

Personally, I practiced the ketogenic diet for half of the year 2018, and I got great benefits from it. I discontinued it since I found it difficult to follow by eating a lot of fruits and vegetables, these being composed of carbohydrates, I could not maintain myself in permanent ketosis. But I am not seriously ill, so my case is not an example here.

In fact I practiced partial ketogenic fasting for a few months, that is to say that I ate almost only fats, and limited my sugar intake to less than 50 grams per day, and I limited the amount of calories to about 1,000 calories a day. Suffice to say that I ate very little in volume, since it represents about 150 grams of food per 24 hours, the fats providing almost 1,000 calories per 100 grams.

In any case from the first day I felt a revival of energy, and the following days it increased again, and I was soon in a state of well-being and dynamism never encountered in my life before!

I could almost have started playing sports! But I just walked the 10,000 steps per day recommended by various authors, and I lost 15 kilos in 6 weeks! And yes, in 1 month and a half I got rid of this overweight which had bothered me for some time already. I lost almost 3 kg a week while having more energy than ever, so I have great memories of this keto-fast!□

Some studies for investigators:

 # 1983-2017 - CHINA STUDY
See the book "The China Study".
Cornell China study https://nutritionstudies.org/the-china-study/

 # 1984 - SEVEN COUNTRIES STUDY
Title: The study of 7 countries: out of 2,289 deaths in 15 years.
https://www.ncbi.nlm.nih.gov/pubmed/6739443 PMID: 6739443

 # 1990 ORNISH - LIFESTYLE HEART TRIAL
Title: Can lifestyle changes reverse coronary heart disease?
The Lancet https://www.ncbi.nlm.nih.gov/pubmed/1973470 PMID: 1973470
"Overall, 82% of the patients in the experimental group had a moderate change towards regression. Comprehensive lifestyle changes can help even severe coronary atherosclerosis, even after just a year, without using lipid-lowering drugs."
Second installment in 1998, translated title: Intensive lifestyle changes to reverse coronary artery disease.
Intensive lifestyle changes for reversal of coronary heart disease. https://www.ncbi.nlm.nih.gov/pubmed/9863851

 # 1992 - 2019 - EPIC STUDY
Source http://epic.iarc.fr/about/background.php
EPIC is the largest epidemiological study on links between food and health never undertaken. Coordinated by the International Agency for Research on Cancer (IARC) of the World Health Organization (WHO), based in Lyon, it relies on a cohort of 521,000 men and women, recruited from 10 European countries: I " Germany, Denmark, Spain, France, Greece, Holland, Italy, Norway, the United Kingdom and Sweden.

 # 1994 - 1999 - LYON HEART STUDY
Title: Mediterranean diet, traditional risk factors and rate of cardiovascular complications after myocardial infarction: final report of the Lyon Diet Heart study. INSERM, Study of Lyon. 1994
https://www.ncbi.nlm.nih.gov/pubmed/7911176?dopt=Abstract
Second installment: Mediterranean diet rich in alpha-linolenic acid in secondary prevention of coronary heart disease. 1999
https://www.ncbi.nlm.nih.gov/pubmed/9989963?dopt=Abstract

 # 2004 - INTERHEART

Title: Effect of potentially modifiable risk factors associated with myocardial infarction in 52 countries (INTERHEART study) : case-control study. https://www.ncbi.nlm.nih.gov/pubmed/15364185 PMID: 15364185

2005 by Dr Cordain
Title: Origins and evolution of the Western diet: health implications for the 21st century. https://www.ncbi.nlm.nih.gov/pubmed/15699220

2009 Arch Intern Med.
Title: A systematic review of the evidence supporting a causal link between dietary factors and coronary heart disease. https://www.ncbi.nlm.nih.gov/pubmed/19364995 PMID: 19364995

2013 - PREDIMED
Title: Primary prevention of cardiovascular disease with a Mediterranean diet. https://www.ncbi.nlm.nih.gov/pubmed/29897867 PMID: 29897867
        "Small diet changes and little adherence control, but still very positive results."

2014 by Dr Vasto
Title: Mediterranean diet and longevity: an example of nutraceuticals? https://www.ncbi.nlm.nih.gov/pubmed/24350926 PMID: 24350926

2015 - MEDHEA STUDY
Title: The Mediterranean diet: health, science and society. https://www.ncbi.nlm.nih.gov/pubmed/26148921 PMID: 26148921

2016 - INTERSTROKE
Title: Global and regional effects of potentially modifiable risk factors associated with acute stroke in 32 countries (INTERSTROKE): a case-control study. https://www.ncbi.nlm.nih.gov/pubmed/27431356 PMID: 27431356

2017 - The Lancet
Title: Coronary atherosclerosis in South American Gypsy natives: a cross-sectional cohort study. https://www.ncbi.nlm.nih.gov/pubmed/28320601 PMID: 28320601

Ideal physical activity

We discovered in the previous chapters the importance of physical activity to be healthy, whether in disease prevention or treatment. Humans have always been active from morning to evening for the past millennia, and this seems essential to the health of the body, which without regular use ends up degrading. Living biology is thus made, what is not used tends to disappear.

It was not until the last century, with the advent of the industrialization of society, that humans locally ceased to be farmers, and became sedentary, and gradually moved away from all physical work. In less developed countries, the population is still much more physically active, living in the countryside and without too much mechanical means of transport, which is definitely a positive factor contributing to their better health. The arduous or intensive work 8 hours a day is not beneficial either, and it is thus necessary to find a balance, where one activates at least 1 or 2 hours per day in an average way, and several times a week more intensely, to the point where our pulse and breathing speed up.

This chapter presents official WHO data on the amount of exercise, as well as summaries of studies, and a very didactic book to learn running. Sports and physical activities are many and varied, take advice from a professional to determine what would be best for you, then make the effort to practice, it is very important for you. Of course the first weeks the body adapts and this can generate discomfort, but then, the body releasing endorphins with pleasant sensations during physical exercise, it becomes a source of pleasure!

From the Senegal Ministry of Health website:
http://www.sante.gouv.sn/
The benefits of sport are legion! Indeed, physical activity allows you to feel good in your body and your head, while having fun. But how often do you exercise? A workout of 30 minutes of physical exercise a day is ideal for healthy living. But note that if you need to / want to lose weight or reach specific goals, you will need to train more.

Sport prevents illnesses and health problems. It stimulates high density lipoproteins (HDL) and lowers the level of triglyceride, the main constituent of fat. Physical activity improves blood circulation, reducing the risk of heart disease. In fact, regular exercise helps prevent health problems such as stroke, metabolic problems, heart attacks, type 2 diabetes, depression, different types of cancer and arthritis.

Exercise makes you cheerful, stimulating various brain chemicals, sport makes you happier and calmer. In addition, sport positively influences self-confidence. Thus, if you train regularly, you will feel better in your body, but also in your head.

Sport increases your energy level. It strengthens your muscles and improves your endurance. Through sport, you oxygenate your muscles and your heart more, allowing your cardiovascular system to work more efficiently. And, if your heart and lungs work better, you will have more energy. Exercise improves sleep. Exercising regularly allows you to fall asleep quickly and sleep more deeply. Please note: it is better to avoid exercising just before diving under the duvet: you cannot sleep!

From the World Health Organization website: https://www.who.int

Information from the 2010 WHO report "Global recommendations for physical activity for health", downloadable for free from their website. ISBN 9789241599979

Too bad they don't offer more recent data, but these quantitative WHO recommendations on physical activity correspond well to what we find in many clinical studies.

Presentation: WHO has developed these global recommendations on physical activity for health with the aim of providing national and regional policy makers with indications on the dose / effect relationship between frequency, duration, intensity , the type and total amount of physical activity needed to prevent non communicable diseases.

These guidelines have been approved by the WHO Guidelines Review Committee. For each age category they offer links that lead to more information.

The recommendations concern three age groups:

From 5 to 17 years of age: For children and young people, physical activity includes play, sports, travel, daily tasks, recreational activities, physical education or the planned exercise, in the family, school or community context. In order to improve their cardio respiratory endurance, their muscular and bone state and the cardiovascular and metabolic biological markers:

1- Children and young people aged 5 to 17 years should accumulate at least 60 minutes per day of physical activity, moderate to sustained intensity.

2- The fact of practicing physical activity for more than 60 minutes brings an additional health benefit.

3- Daily physical activity should be essentially an endurance activity. Sustained activities, especially those that strengthen the muscular system and bone condition, should be incorporated at least three times a week.

18 to 64 years old: For adults aged 18 to 64, physical activity includes leisure, travel (for example walking or cycling), professional activities, household chores, play activities, sports or planned exercise, in daily, family or community context. In order to improve their cardiorespiratory endurance, their muscular and bone condition, and to reduce the risk of non-communicable diseases and depression:

1- Adults aged 18 to 64 should practice at least 150 minutes during the week moderate intensity endurance activity or at least 75 minutes of sustained intensity endurance activity, or an equivalent combination of moderate and sustained intensity activity.

2- The endurance activity should be practiced in periods of at least 10 minutes.

3- In order to obtain additional health benefits, adults should increase the duration of their moderate intensity endurance activity to reach 300 minutes per week or practice 150 minutes per week of physical activity. endurance of sustained intensity, or an equivalent combination of activity of moderate and sustained intensity.

4- Muscle strengthening exercises involving the main muscle groups should be practiced at least two days a week.

From 65 years and over: For people aged 65 and over, physical activity includes leisure, travel (for example walking or cycling), professional activities, household chores, play activities, sports or planned exercise, in the daily, family or community context. In order to improve their cardiorespiratory endurance, their muscular and bone condition, and to reduce the risk of noncommunicable diseases, depression and deterioration of cognitive function:

1- Elderly people should practice at least, during the week, 150 minutes of moderate intensity endurance activity or at least 75 minutes of sustained intensity endurance activity, or an equivalent combination of moderate and sustained intensity activity.

2- The endurance activity should be practiced in periods of at least 10 minutes.

3- In order to benefit from additional health benefits, the elderly should increase the duration of their moderate intensity endurance activity so as to reach 300 minutes per week or practice 150 minutes per week of activity. sustained intensity endurance, or an equivalent combination of moderate and sustained intensity activity.

4- Elderly people with reduced mobility should practice physical activity aimed at improving balance and preventing falls at least three days a week.

5- Muscle strengthening exercises involving the main muscle groups should be done at least two days a week.

6- When elderly people cannot exercise the recommended amount of physical activity due to their state of health, they should be as physically active as their abilities and condition allow.

A study that concludes that the positive effects on blood circulation and respiration, of 8 days of the Mediterranean Diet combined with physical exercises, are still present after 1 year.

"Cardio. MedDiet. Long-term effects of an exercise and Mediterranean diet intervention in the vascular function of an older, healthy population. 2014"
https://www.ncbi.nlm.nih.gov/pubmed/25109875/
BACKGROUND: Preserving endothelial function and microvascular integrity is suggested to reduce the risk of cardiovascular disease. It has recently been shown that the age-dependent decline in endothelial and microvascular integrity can be reversed by combining exercise with a Mediterranean diet (MD) in an 8-week intervention. The present study examines whether the improvement in risk reduction in microcirculatory and cardiorespiratory functions is maintained in this age group after one year of follow-up.

DESIGN AND METHODS: Twenty healthy sedentary participants (55 years ± 4 years) of the original study underwent a cardiopulmonary exercise tolerance test and were evaluated for their endothelial cutaneous vascular conductance of the upper and lower limbs (CVC) in using Doppler laser fluximetry (LDF) with dependent endothelium [ACh (acetylcholine chloride)] and endothelium-independent vasodilation (SNP (sodium nitroprusside)), 1 year after the end of the intervention.

CONCLUSIONS: Initial improvements from an 8-week exercise and MD intervention were still evident, particularly in microcirculatory and cardiorespiratory assessments, 1 year after the initial study. This suggests that a brief intervention combining MD and exercise in this high-risk group promises long-term health benefits.

And a study on the essential importance of physical exercise. "Physical activity - the Holy Grail of modern medicine?" 2017.
https://www.ncbi.nlm.nih.gov/pubmed/29127758
Abstract: Movement is the basic attribute of life. It is not surprising that returning to regular physical activity is a very effective and inexpensive way to prevent and treat most noncommunicable diseases.

Therefore, each physician should be able to prescribe appropriate physical activity. The minimum amount of physical activity with proven effects in primary prevention of chronic disease is relatively low: 150 minutes of moderate physical activity or 75 minutes of high intensity exercise per week or a combination of both.

The easiest and safest way to get physical activity is to walk (at least 10,000 steps / day or 6,000 steps / day in addition to daily activities).

The FITT model is a more sophisticated way of prescribing a physical activity that already requires a stress test. Patients at risk for atherosclerosis or with any manifestation of atherosclerosis (patients with coronary artery disease, post-stroke, peripheral arterial disease) benefit from exercise as well as patients with chronic heart failure.

Physical activity also helps patients with lung diseases (COPD, asthma), metabolic diseases (diabetes mellitus, obesity, osteoporosis) and also rheumatic diseases. Regular exercise improves cognitive function, reduces depression and anxiety, and helps addicts. Recently, exercise has also been shown to alter the gut microbiome. One of the mechanisms that contribute to the beneficial effect of exercise is what are called "exercise factors" - myokines.

Physical activity, when properly prescribed, is an inexpensive and universal medication with minimal side effects. It is our "home pharmacy" that we always have with us.□

Taking action

This last part of the book aims to keep on hand the key points verified by these doctors. Of course, each of them gives many details and additional recommendations in their respective books, which I invite you to read, to buy but also to offer around you, out of compassion for your loved ones.

Food action

Regarding the right way to eat, these medical professionals all recommend eating foods the least processed possible, in the form that nature gives them. So let's eat raw fruits and vegetables when possible, and cook gently for legumes and whole grains, and to warm us up as needed.

Foods recommended by all these doctors (to eat as much as possible):

The staple food of still healthy populations is vegetable. It includes all raw edible fruits and vegetables, legumes, beans, lentils, sweet potatoes that require gentle cooking.

In these populations, including in the traditional Mediterranean, animal products are present in small quantities to give taste, and not daily.

Foods Rejected by Dr. Seignalet and Dr. Greger:

Dairy Products.

Foods rejected only by Dr. Seignalet:

Cereals, even whole, apart from rice and buckwheat.

Cooking

The Mediterranean traditionally cooks little and especially with steam and slowly. This is also what these doctors recommend, since many essential micronutrients and enzymes are destroyed at higher temperatures.

The worst being grilled meats and fried foods which also produce carcinogenic toxins and denature the proteins which are then harmful, especially with animal products.

Drinks:

Very sweet fruit or vegetable juices are not recommended, as it is mainly sugary water, which will cause a strong spike in blood sugar. The fruits will be eaten whole, with their fibers which slow down the absorption of sugars. Fruits are not eaten abundantly in healthy populations, the most important seems to be vegetables and legumes.

Green or slightly sweet leafy vegetable juices are recommended for people who want to speed up the remineralization of their bodies. Indeed 500 ml of fresh green juice in the day can provide a very large number of micronutrients and minerals and trace elements, which will be quickly absorbed into the blood.

Alcohol is considered harmful in all cases, by all these doctors, with the exception of Dr. de Lorgeril who considers that red wine during the meal brings benefits, which he unfortunately could not test during the study of Lyon, for ethical reasons.

Soft drinks are considered harmful by all these doctors, by their high concentration of fast sugars, but perhaps especially by their high content of dissolved CO_2 (the gas that makes up the bubbles), since this gas is acidifying on contact with water. It is well known that the oceans acidify with the absorption of CO_2 present in the atmosphere, which benefits pathogenic microorganisms which are present in acidic environment. Our body is made up of more than 65% of water, and we exhale CO_2 during the breathing process, so it seems paradoxical to ingest it artificially.

The books to take action:
Eating Mediterranean:
The new Mediterranean diet - Dr. Michel Lorgevil - 2020 - ISBN 978-2501150293
Eating hypotoxic:
"Understanding and practicing Seignalet regime" - Dominique Seignalet - 2014 - ISBN 978-2755405637
Eating Paleo:
"The Paleo diet: The diet without processed foods to get into shape" - Dr. Loren Cordain - 2015 - ISBN 978-2013964548
Eating ketogenic:
"Long live ketogenic food!" - Dr. Alexandra Dalu - 2016 - ISBN 979-1028501983
Eating against dementia:
"Curing Alzheimer: Understand and act in time" - Dr. Michael Nehls - 2017 - ISBN 978-2330072834
Remineralization with green juice:
"The benefits of vegetables and fruit juices" - Kara Rosen - 2015 - ISBN 978-2035905772
Remineralization with seawater:
"Quinton: The serum of life" - Jean-Claude Rodet, Maxence Layet - 2008 - ISBN 978-2702906378

Action collagen and supplements

Supplementation for collagen

Collagen is the basis for the constitution of our body, we must ensure to give it the elements necessary for its manufacture. Mainly you have to make sure you have enough vitamin C, lysine and proline.

A high daily consumption of fresh fruits and vegetables provides good doses of vitamin C.

Lysine is one of the essential amino acids, that is to say that it must be ingested because the body cannot manufacture it. Products rich in lysine are eggs, red meats, cod and sardines, and some legumes (beans, peas and lentils), dairy products and soy.

Proline can be produced by the body, but less and less with age.

According to some of these doctors, the amounts of vitamin C (ascorbic acid) and lysine absorbed with food are insufficient, as well as the endogenous production of proline, and they recommend taking vitamin C supplements, from 3 to 6 grams per day for a healthy adult, and more when sick, and 3 to 6 grams of lysine and proline per day. Vitamin C has a life of 1/2 hour in the body, it is better to take it several times a day, rather than just once.

This practice, developed by Dr Rath and Pauling (see their joint patent), is known on the internet as "Pauling Therapy". Some American sites offer this formula in the form of powder or tablets, making it easier to take these 3 elements in large doses. We are advised to take 3 doses per day, each containing about 1 gram of each of the 3 elements, or 3 grams of each per day. Personally I take it as soon as I have the opportunity!

There are also several kinds of collagen supplements, some of which appear to have positive effects on painful joints, according to several published clinical studies. Most are made from animal gelatin, the collagen hydrolyzate. But beware, many cheap offers are poor quality products from animal carcasses. Some studies used 10 mg or less of undenatured type 2 collagen (UC-II) per day, others used 10 grams of collagen hydrolyzate (CH-Alpha).

Supplementation for alpha lipoic acid

Dr. Schwartz advises taking alpha lipoic acid as part of his "metabolic treatment" against cancer, which is taken with conventional treatments. See his books or consult them for dosages, as it is ineffective against cancer if taken alone.

The dosage he mentions is 800 mg in the morning and 800 mg in the evening of alpha-lipoic acid, with 500 mg in the morning, noon and evening of hydroxycitrate. If you take hydroxycitrate in the form of Garcinia Cambogia capsules, then you have to go up to 800 mg per dose, since this extract often contains only 60% of hydroxycitrate.

There are capsules of alpha lipoic acid on the internet, between 15 and 30 euros for 120 capsules. The same goes for hydroxycitrate.

The books to take action:
To supplement with Vitamin C:

"Healing with vitamin C: Diseases treated, beneficial effects, types, modes of administration." - Stefano Pravato - 2016 - ISBN 978-8862298001

"Why animals don't have a heart attack… men do!" - Dr. Matthias Rath - 2009 - ISBN 978-9076332550

To supplement with lipoic acid and hydroxy-citrate:

"Cancer: A simple, non-toxic treatment" - Dr. Lawrence Schwartz, 2016, ISBN 978-2365491778

☐

Action physical activity

This is the easiest part to explain, since it comes down to moving enough.
This information can be found here
https://www.who.int/dietphysicalactivity/factsheet_recommendations/en/

Minimum amount of physical activity recommended by the WHO:
Adults aged 18 to 64 should practice at least, during the week, 150 minutes of moderate intensity endurance activity or at least 75 minutes of sustained intensity endurance activity, or an equivalent combination of moderate and sustained intensity activity.

Endurance activity should be practiced in periods of at least 10 minutes.

In order to gain additional health benefits, adults should increase the duration of their moderate intensity endurance activity to 300 minutes per week or exercise 150 minutes per week of endurance activity of intense intensity, or an equivalent combination of activity of moderate and sustained intensity.

Muscle building exercises involving the major muscle groups should be done at least two days a week. "
This can result in:
At a minimum:

30 min per day of moderate physical exercise, such as walking, swimming or cycling, 5 times a week.

Plus 4 times 20 minutes of intensive activities per week.
And to really get the best health benefits, you have to double that:

1 hour of moderate exercise 5 times a week
Plus 4 times 40 minutes of intensive activity per week.

We then realize how far the majority of humans in industrialized countries are far from it! Because we can find a lot of people who walk 1 hour a day, but we are little to add to that 4 sessions per week of intensive exercise!

For chronic or long-term sedentary people, or the sick, consult your doctor to know your initial physical capacity and your contraindications, then refer to sports professionals, as in sports halls, to guide you to departure, because at the beginning it is not obvious to practice reasonably and correctly, any sport that it is.

And stick to it, you may progress slowly, but surely!

Action Pollution

All these doctors are unanimous, smoking must stop to prevent these serious diseases, because it is very toxic for our cells.

Dr. Schwartz, who has conducted studies on the toxicity of cigarettes, has discovered that the most dangerous is absorbed CO_2, rather than tar. Tobacco companies stopped funding his research once he found the real cause of the danger of smoking, and even after he figured out how to prevent it ... why?

Air pollution was already causing serious problems for people who heat themselves with wood, then coal, then in areas where industries developed.

But nothing compares to the burning by our hundreds of millions of vehicles, mixtures of hydrocarbons and multiple synthetic molecules, which release them right under our noses, in the middle of the places where we live!

Then add the chemicals that have been developed for the industrialization of agriculture, the many chemicals sprayed in the air or spread, and found in soil, water and food ...

The best advice in the field of prevention of these toxic pollutants, is either to live with a permanent filtering mask, or to go to live in the countryside, or at least in an area little polluted, for example thanks to the regular winds which clean its air, and where chemical agriculture is little present.

It is unfortunately the least easy part to implement to protect oneself, since being outside our direct power of influence.

Against pollution, it is the concept of industrial society and massive consumption that must be changed. Or finally put in place existing recycling solutions, and manufacturing processes that respect the environment and our biology.

These pollutions, which are harmful to our health, are the responsibility of political decision-makers and shareholders of industries. Let us make them aware of the massive poisoning in which they participate!

Stress / Sleep Action

Stress management is very important, because it causes chemical reactions that end up damaging our body when it becomes chronic.

A little punctual stress, like during physical activities, is necessary and beneficial, but permanent stress, even mental, is toxic. Sleep is also very important for staying healthy, and it improves when you start to do physical activities, which is very beneficial. You have to make sure you orient your life in such a way that you fall asleep easily at night, and that you spend peaceful and restful nights.

Food is very important in this area too, both food and drink.

The books to take action:
Relaxing with meditation:
"The art of meditation" - Matthieu Ricard - 2010 - ISBN 978-2266194242
Soften psychological trauma:
"EMDR" - Dr Jacques Roques - 2016 - ISBN 978-2130730033□

Thank you for taking the time to read me, good luck and good health!

Find all my information on the internet: www.veryveryhealthy.com

This book was written in France
Legal deposit paper book in French: February 2020

www.ingramcontent.com/pod-product-compliance
Lightning Source LLC
LaVergne TN
LVHW051224200726
843510LV00011B/1472